Essent in Pati̶ Care

Edited by

K.W.M. Fulford
Steven Ersser
Tony Hope

b

**Blackwell
Science**

© 1996 by
Blackwell Science Ltd
Chapter 1 © 1996 by K.W.M. Fulford
Editorial Offices:
Osney Mead, Oxford OX2 0EL
25 John Street, London WC1N 2BL
23 Ainslie Place, Edinburgh EH3 6AJ
238 Main Street, Cambridge
  Massachusetts 02142, USA
54 University Street, Carlton
  Victoria 3053, Australia

Other Editorial Offices:
Arnette Blackwell SA
  1, rue de Lille, 75007 Paris
  France

Blackwell Wissenschafts-Verlag GmbH
  Kurfürstendamm 57
  10707 Berlin, Germany

Feldgasse 13, A-1238 Wien
Austria

First published 1996

Set in 10/12 pt Palatino
by DP Photosetting, Aylesbury, Bucks
Printed and bound in Great Britain
by Hartnolls Ltd., Bodmin, Cornwall

DISTRIBUTORS

Marston Book Services Ltd
PO Box 87
Oxford OX2 0DT
(*Orders:* Tel: 01865 791155
      Fax: 01865 791927
      Telex: 837515)

North America
Blackwell Science, Inc.
238 Main Street
Cambridge, MA 02142
(*Orders:* Tel: 800 215-1000
            617 876-7000
      Fax: 617 492-5263)

Australia
Blackwell Science Pty Ltd
54 University Street
Carlton, Victoria 3053
(*Orders:* Tel: 03 347-0300
      Fax: 03 349-3016)

A catalogue record for this title
is available from the British Library

ISBN 0–632–03903–5

Library of Congress
Cataloging-in-Publication Data

Essential practice in patient-centred care/
  edited by K.W.M. Fulford,
  Steven Ersser, Tony Hope.
      p.   cm.
    Includes bibliographical references
  and index.
    ISBN 0–632–03903–5 (alk. paper)
    1. Medical personnel and patient.
  I. Fulford, K.W.M.   II. Ersser, Steven.
  III. Hope, R.A.
    [DNLM: 1. Patient-Centered Care.
  2. Patient Participation. W
  84.5 E78 1996]
  R727.3.E86   1995
  362.1—dc20
  DNLM/DLC
  for Library of Congress   95-35999
                                      CIP

Contents

List of Contributors

Ann Bradshaw   SRN, DipN (Lond), PhD, Macmillan Lecturer in Palliative Nursing, National Institute for Nursing, Oxford.

Margaret Brazier   LLB, Barrister, Professor of Law, University of Manchester.

Ruth Chadwick   BPhil, MA, DPhil (Oxon), LLB (London), Professor of Moral Philosophy, Head of Centre for Professional Ethics, University of Central Lancashire.

Roger Crisp   BPhil, MA, DPhil, Fellow and Tutor in Philosophy, St Anne's College, Oxford.

John Devereux   BA (Qld), LLB (Qld), DPhil (Oxford), Barrister of the Supreme Court of Queensland, Senior Lecturer in Law and Deputy Dean of the Faculty of Law, Griffith University, Queensland, Australia.

Len Doyal   BA, MSc, Reader in Medical Ethics, The London and St Bartholomew's Hospitals Medical Colleges, University of London.

Maeve Ennis   BA, Lecturer in Health Psychology, University College, London.

Steven Ersser   BSc (Hons), RGN, Senior Lecturer/Research Associate, School of Health Care Studies, Oxford Brookes University, former Fellow, National Institute for Nursing, Oxford.

Martyn Evans   BA, PhD, University College Fellow, Centre for Philosophy and Health Care, University of Wales, Swansea.

Ray Fitzpatrick   BA, MSc, PhD, (Hon) MFPHM, Fellow, Nuffield College, Oxford and University Lecturer in Medical Sociology, University of Oxford.

K.W.M. (Bill) Fulford   DPhil (Oxon), FRCPsych, Professor of Philosophy and Mental Health, Department of Philosophy, University of Warwick, and Director, Oxford Practice Skills Programme, Medical School, Oxford.

John Hall   BA, MSc, PhD, C Psychol, FBPsS, Professional Adviser in Clinical Psychology, Oxfordshire National Health Service Trusts, and Honorary Senior Clinical Lecturer, University of Oxford.

Christopher Heginbotham   BSc, MSc, MA, Chief Executive, Riverside Mental Health Trust, London.

Roger Higgs   MBE, MA, FRCP, FRCGP, General Practitioner and Professor, Department of General Practice and Primary Care, King's College School of Medicine, London.

Tony Hope   MA, PhD, MBBS, MRCPsych, Lecturer in Practice Skills, University of Oxford, and Honorary Consultant Psychiatrist.

Steven F. Horowitz   MD, Chief, Division of Cardiology, and Medical Director, The Samuels Planetree Model Hospital Unit, Beth Israel Medical Center,

New York and Professor of Medicine and Nuclear Medicine, Albert Einstein College of Medicine, New York.

Peter Jarvis   BD, BA (Econ), MSocSc, PhD, FRSA, Professor of Continuing Education and Head of Department, Department of Educational Studies, University of Surrey.

Mary Judge   Non-executive Director, Oxford Radcliffe Hospital NHS Trust, and former Chair, Community Health Council, Oxfordshire.

Alison Kitson   BSc (Hons), DPhil, RGN, FRCN, Director, National Institute of Nursing, Oxford, Acting Principal, RCN Institute.

Sally M.A. Lloyd-Bostock   BA, DPhil, BA, Research Fellow, Centre for Socio-Legal Studies, Oxford University.

Andrew C. Markus   MA, BMBCh, FRCGP, MRCP, Emeritus Fellow, Green College, Oxford, General Practitioner (retired), Thame, Oxfordshire.

Trevor Martin   BA, BArch, RIBA, Partner, CODA Architects, Bristol.

Donald McIntyre   MA, MEd, Reader in Educational Studies, University of Oxford.

Shirley McIver   BSc (Hons), PhD, Senior Fellow, Health Services Management Centre, University of Birmingham.

David W. Millard   MA, MD, FRCPsych, Emeritus Fellow, Green College, Oxford.

Jonathan Montgomery   BA, LLM, Senior Lecturer in Law, University of Southampton.

Linda Mulcahy   LLB, LLM (Legal theory), Lawford Reader in Public Law, University of North London.

Ruth Ravich   BA, Director, Patient Representative Department, Mount Sinai Medical Center, New York.

F.D. Rose   BSc, PhD, C Psychol, FBPsS, Professor of Psychology, University of East London.

Terence Ryan   DM, FRCP, Clinical Professor of Dermatology, Oxford Radcliffe Hospital, The Churchill, Oxford.

Lucy Schmolka   MA (Health Advocacy), Patient Representative, Mount Sinai Medical Center, New York.

Veronica J. Thomas   RGN, DipN, BSc, PhD, C Psychol, Senior Research Fellow, Department of Nursing Studies, Kings College, London University.

Angie Titchen   MCSP, MSc, Research and Development Fellow, National Institute for Nursing, Oxford.

Stephen Graham Wright   MBE, RGN, DipN, RCNT, DANS, RNT, MSc (Nursing), MHSM, FRCN, Director, The European Nursing Development Agency (TENDA) Lancashire, and Visiting Professor of Nursing, University of Southampton.

Perspectives on Patient-Centred Care

A Patient's Perspective

Mary Judge

Most members of the general public will not have been aware that there could be any other than care centred around the patient. If health care is not about the patient, who is it about ... the convenience of the consultant, the training of the junior nurse, the rota of the porters? Perhaps a realistic view is that it is a mixture of all of these. The quality of care for the patient would suffer if staff were not able to give of their best endeavours because the world around did not function efficiently.

This book is written to clarify and explain the professional aspects of patient-centred care and to discuss how the many people involved could improve the care of the individual patient. It brings together the work of a remarkable range of practitioners and researchers who have contributed in different ways to patient centredness, illustrating the significance of their individual disciplines, and showing clearly – through critical cross-disciplinary commentaries – how modern health care depends crucially on these disciplines working together.

Health is a big issue for all of us. As people become more aware of their own responsibilities for their own health there is increased interaction between clinician and patient. The medical media play their part in this through the deluge of information ranging from wild conjecture to reasoned discussion of the latest research findings. Outcomes are part of the debate and questions are being asked. For the interested layman the clouds which have hung round the choice of treatment are now beginning to clear, as people are encouraged to take informed decisions about their own treatment with as much help as they need.

Patients need to feel confident enough to ask questions, to go to a consultation with a notebook and to use the nurse as communicator and advocate. So the move towards putting the patient into the centre of planning for services may represent more than the changes (important as they are) in environment, in equipment, and in professional attitudes, which are the subject of this book. What is involved is a whole new way of looking at health care.

Traditional attitudes from the near past are still very much around, and there are many who look back sadly to the demise of the all powerful matron, without seeing the changes in nursing which are an integral part of the move towards patient-centred care, and which have led to the 'named nurse' as someone who knows about individual treatment and care. The benevolent doctor, who did not worry his patients with the treatment he would prescribe, took comforting responsibility for their health, and so saved them from a great deal of anxiety and stress. People stayed in hospital until all bodily functions were working and there was little to be done at home except to convalesce. Time is running out for this thinking, and that may be all to the good. Hospitals can be dangerous places to be in for too long for those whose resistance to infection is low.

It is of course very easy to talk about 'the public' as though everyone has similar needs and aspirations. In fact not only are their needs different, but the way people react to situations may be very different; planners, purchasers and providers of services must acknowledge this. But the public can be divided into identifiable groups:

- The direct user of the services – sitting in the GP's waiting room, in out-patients, on a trolley in accident and emergency, occupying a bed on the ward.
- The carer – a relative, neighbour or friend – who is likely to feel responsible for the patient when he or she leaves hospital, and who rightly has a much higher profile than in the past. Some of these carers act as proxy for those unable to speak for themselves – the very old and the very young, as well as for those with difficulty in communicating.
- All of us who are potential users of health services for whom the planning and provision make for a better or worse lifestyle.

Public expectations are changing very fast. Clinicians are able to cure or alleviate more conditions, and miracles happen every day. And yet public anxiety persists, and manifests itself in rising levels of complaints. Somehow the pace at which change is happening makes for unease, and we do not feel ready to take on the additional responsibility for the care not only of ourselves but of our families. The move towards a patient-centred approach could help to support and educate everyone.

Ill people are not always best placed to evaluate their experience of being in hospital. They feel, and indeed are, dependent on those caring for them and have no standard for comparison. In many cases they may not understand the implication of what is being done to them until they have time to think later. There is enormous scope for the practitioners to explore with the patient their experience of their illness.

The system of complaints has been fair neither to the patients nor to the staff. Confusion and lack of response left the complainant feeling bruised and unhappy, with the medical profession ranged against them. Staff felt that they were unfairly threatened. The new guidelines on complaints accepted by the minister in March 1995 should help to reduce the problem. However there is much scope for individual trusts to make it easier for patients to communicate with them. There is plenty of evidence, from community health councils and others, that the motivation of the majority of patients who complain is to improve the service, and to prevent the same thing happening to someone else.

The move towards a simplified complaints system should, I believe, give people the confidence to feel that they can talk about their anxieties to those who are able to help.

Clinicians are working hard to reduce the length of stays in hospital. Some of this effort is designed to use resources wisely where patients do not need specialist care; in many cases it allows the patient to get where they want to be – at home. The winter crises, which have affected general hospitals all over the country, are now seen as part of a more general pattern of increasing need for health care. With fewer beds in the system this increasing need puts immense pressure on the carers who support those coming out of hospital. More and more people do not have anyone who is able or willing to look after them, and community help must inevitably go to them. But this puts a heavy burden on the carers which they may be unhappy to assume, and for which they may sometimes feel that they have no training and little aptitude.

There is a need for education which starts when the patient and the carer are in contact with the hospital and in the care of multi-professionals. Such education would embrace recognizing symptoms, understanding when things are getting serious, knowing how to give drugs and recognizing their side effects, and above all learning how to lift and move without doing damage. The opportunity to promote a healthy lifestyle is increasingly seen as part of acute care. The awareness that cycling saves time, that exercise makes you feel good, and that the food that is good for you happens to be the food you enjoy, are all encouraging signs of the times.

For the potential user of the NHS there is more openness about its services than ever before. There is very little about the planning and running of services which is not already in the public domain if people want the information, although the sheer volume of information available is daunting. The information is indeed abundant: figures about outcomes, figures about funding, figures about where the money is spent and, above all, figures on the standards achieved. A new commitment to making people aware of outcomes and the effectiveness of treatments will guide the research and development programmes. 'Does this treatment for varicose veins work, what are the available data, what are the chances of failure, what happens if I elect to have it done?' Patients are increasingly making informed decisions about the treatment they want, for conditions ranging from their child's glue ear to heart transplants.

The importance of all this is that the body in the bed and the carer sitting alongside are becoming progressively better informed and are beginning, with the help of professionals, to take more responsibility for their own health, and to have the confidence to choose a preferred outcome, when that is appropriate. The practical effect of the patient-centred approach will be to encourage and support patients and carers to learn from their experience. It is a powerful challenge to the professionals who are driving this initiative in the best interests of the patient – a challenge which this book will help them meet.

A Nurse's Perspective

Alison Kitson

It is often the case that one is required to reconsider those taken-for-granted essential elements of one's practice when faced with rapid change. And it is certainly the case that in today's health care system, in every country, in every continent in the world, policy makers, politicians and professionals are being challenged to redefine the parameters of health care. Both the context in which care is delivered and the ideological basis upon which it has developed are changing.

New roles, new boundaries and transformation in patients' expectations and attitudes to health care have changed the context of care. Changes in junior doctors' roles impact upon senior medical roles, and boundaries with nursing and other staff are profoundly changing the delivery of health care. The shift in emphasis from hospital-based to primary health care is also having a big effect on how doctors and nurses deliver a service to patients. Add to this the constant requirement to contain costs and one has a picture of a service having to cope with ever increasing demand within financial constraints, and providers struggling to deliver an adequate, safe, cost effective, humane service.

Whether one can call it a caring or indeed a patient-centred service is surely becoming a moot point. The ideological base of universal coverage, care from the cradle to the grave as epitomized in the 1948 NHS legislation, is becoming increasingly difficult to realize. The philosophy of doctors and nurses being called to a special vocation to serve their community is also beginning to be challenged. With the increasing emphasis on evidence-based health care, clinical and cost effectiveness, are we not in danger of forgetting about the human being who also happens to present with a treatable condition?

There is possibly no more important a time than now to explore those core beliefs and values that define for us what is essential in the way we look after the sick, frail, vulnerable, confused, depressed, anxious and disadvantaged. The fact that we make assumptions regarding our own understanding of the link between clinical competence, compassion, caring and our ability to communicate with patients is clearly brought out in several of the chapter contributions. Our ability to grasp colleagues' perspectives is equally suspect and our heroic failures to understand the patient's view are constantly brought to our attention.

How then can a book on essential practice in patient-centred care help us to see things more clearly? First, it explores the assumptions and beliefs we all hold about the way we give care. Whether we have trained as a doctor, nurse or physiotherapist, we base our understanding of the human dimension of caring on such things as experience, belief and what the system permits. When none of these dimensions is defined explicitly, and particularly when other stronger forces come into play, then quite major shifts can occur in our behaviour and consequently in our attitudes and values. To explore such underlying values and beliefs is essential to patient-centred practice.

Second, we need to understand the patient experience in much more detail. We need to remind ourselves of the fears, worries and concerns that patients experience; their frustration at losing autonomy over parts of their lives and their need to negotiate new relationships with professionals supposedly 'on their side'. Just having time to talk or to be with a patient is becoming increasingly difficult in today's cost conscious health care system. What will happen if doctors and nurses stop engaging with their patients? Would it matter that much or would we be praised for reaching financial targets and improving throughput?

The constant frustration for many nurses is the lack of time they have to be with their patients. Until such functions as support, reassurance, comfort and caring can be quantified it seems that policy makers and managers do not value and therefore do not fund them. Do we have to prove their value from a clinical, scientific base or can we declare them as basic rights for every patient, and as such ought they to be the foundation stones of professional education and evaluations of the quality of patient care? Are patients allowed the time to be sick any more and, equally pertinent, are they permitted time to recover?

There is no professional territoriality when it comes to compassion, justice and respect for persons. We the professionals become as much victims of the system as our patients if we do not take responsibility for ensuring patient-centred care. The only difference is that we, the professionals, labour under the illusion of being free from the effect of a health care system that has lost sight of its ultimate goal which, I believe, is to promote humane, patient-centred care. Yet we too are the losers.

A General Practitioner's Perspective

Andrew Markus

Patient-centred. Multidisciplinary. The buzz words of a few years ago are becoming clichés of the present.

So why do we need yet another look at patient-centred health care? One answer, I think, lies in the increasing alienation of the general public from mainstream medicine. Even fifty years ago, health care was able to offer mainly care, whether by doctors, nurses or others. Cure was at the whim of nature. Then came the technological revolution, with the advent of antibiotic and other curative drugs, and the development of investigative and surgical techniques which make us all marvel. But the concentration on technical procedures has shifted the focus of health care away from the personal interaction of professional with patient.

The growing dissatisfaction of the public with this less personal and apparently less caring situation has become manifest in various ways. It has encouraged the growth and increasing utilization of complementary medicine in all its forms and an ambivalent attitude to mainstream medicine – at once higher expectations and less faith in its delivery. It has also led to increasing complaints by the public against health professionals, and to a rapid growth in the frequency of litigation.

These trends are also seen in countries which spend a much larger proportion of their resources than the UK on health care. Why has this happened at a time when we can perform amazing transplant surgery, fragment internal stones with ultrasound, clear blocked coronary arteries with non-invasive radiologically controlled procedures and so on? This book casts some light on the answers to this question and what can be done to remedy the situation.

In the UK over 95% of doctor–patient contact takes place in a primary care setting. This is the 'coal face' of medical care. Vocational training for general practitioners in the UK has, in recent years, reflected the importance of doctor–patient communication by focusing much teaching on this area. This involves young doctors learning to identify fully what problems have brought patients to seek help, how to use language which patients can understand, and how to make sure that patients have enough information about their illnesses to be able to make informed decisions regarding management.

But it is not enough for this approach to be taught just in primary care. All health professionals need these skills. They need to be taught to students. And those already practising need reminding that we are here to answer patients' needs, not to tell them what to do. The delivery of health care involves many people, from architects who design buildings which make patients and staff feel comfortable, to managers who help staff fulfil their roles. This is what patient-centred care is about, and why this book is important and timely.

Acknowledgements

Several chapters from this book were first presented as papers at a conference organized by the Editors on Patient-Centred Health Care at Green College in Oxford. We are grateful to Green College for the hospitality extended to us on that occasion, and to our many colleagues and friends who have contributed to the development of this book.

I ◆ *The Definition of Patient-Centred Care*

1 ◆ Concepts of Disease and the Meaning of Patient-Centred Care

K.W.M. Fulford

The movement towards patient-centred health care is now well established on a broad front. It encompasses a wide range of both academic and practical disciplines. It is built into medical law and health service administration. Indeed, it has become so much part of the scenery that we hardly stop to ask what patient-centredness in health care really amounts to. There is a sense, after all, in which health care has always been patient-centred. What *is* health care, if not care *of and for* patients? Something has changed, then. There is something 'in the air'. But what is it?

There is no single answer to this question. There is a patient-centredness of nursing (Chapters 6 and 12); another of architecture (Chapter 10); yet others of law (Chapter 9) and management (Chapter 8); another of patient groups and representatives (Chapter 5); and so on. This diversity of disciplines represents a rich resource: the resource of the multi-disciplinary team. A central message of this multi-disciplinary book is that patient-centred care is essentially a co-operative enterprise. But in diversity there is also a danger of confusion. Indeed without a unifying ethic, without a deeper understanding of what is meant by patient-centredness, there is a danger that instead of co-operation between disciplines there will be competition, perhaps even outright conflict, with 'the patient' inevitably the loser.

The focus of this chapter, then, will be the meaning of patient-centred care. Of course, even this narrowed-down question could be approached in a number of ways. Important among these are the ethnographic, participative and other qualitative research methods illustrated later in this book (Chapters 4 and 12). The approach described in this chapter, however, although complementary to these methods (see 'Reading guide'), is, rather, philosophical. Philosophy offers a set of skills for the analysis of concepts (Fulford, 1990). These skills are important to us in health care because different ways of understanding our key guiding concepts, such as illness and disease, may lead to different, and sometimes incompatible, practices.

This has certainly been the case with patient- centred care. As we will see, important differences of understanding have developed between, on the one hand, those concerned with 'patient power', and on the other hand the traditional medical model. In particular, where the patient power movement has emphasized the patient's *values*, the medical model has focused on objective scientific *facts*; and where the patient power movement has emphasized the patient's experience of *illness*, the medical model has emphasized underlying theories of *disease*.

These differences have often been portrayed as differences between patient-centred and doctor-centred care. It would be easy to take sides, but the divide is a false divide, alienating patients and health care professionals alike. The aim of this chapter will thus be to outline a new model, one which incorporates both perspectives. It does displace 'the doctor', or at any rate the hospital specialist, from her traditional pivotal place. At the same time though, it endorses rather than devalues the role of science in health care. It is a model of this kind, incorporating values *and* facts, the lived experience of illness *and* scientific knowledge of disease, which it will be argued is required for genuinely patient-centred health care.

Themes of patient power

The pervasiveness of the patient power movement is impressive. In its most obvious manifestation it is a social and political movement organized into patient groups such as The National Alliance for the Mentally Ill (NAMI) and the Mental Health Association (MHA) in the USA, and, in the UK, The Patients Association and MIND (The National Association for Mental Health).

The movement is also reflected in developments in a number of professional and academic disciplines. Here the most dramatic example is the appearance of an entirely new discipline: bioethics. Born of the tyrannies of an increasingly technological medicine, the clarion call of bioethics has been autonomy, patient *self*-rule against the rule of the doctor (Beauchamp & Childress 1989). There are, as two of the contributors to this book argue, both theological (Chapter 2) and philosophical (Chapter 3) reasons for believing that autonomy is too narrow a principle for health care ethics. This will also be one of the conclusions of the present chapter. Moreover, autonomy and technology are not necessarily incompatible; they may indeed be highly complementary, as in the case of patient-controlled analgesia (Chapter 7). But as a principle, autonomy has been and remains an important bulwark against the worst excesses of medical paternalism. And as a principle supporting patient power, it is one to which a wide range of disciplines have subscribed.

Through all the diversity of the patient power movement, however, there are important unifying themes, both positive and negative. Among positive themes, perhaps the most important of all is an emphasis on *values*. This is the very *raison d'être* of bioethics. But the value-laden nature of medical practice has been strongly emphasized also by other disciplines, in particular by sociologists working on the features by which illness is marked out from other negatively evaluated experiences (Lockyer 1981; Sedgwick 1973); by philosophers (Agich 1983; Reich 1991); and above all, by patients themselves (Toombs 1993; Rogers *et al.* 1993).

This ties in closely with a second positive theme: that the patient's immediate experience of illness is as important as the doctor's more theoretical knowledge of underlying disease processes. Again this is manifest in various ways: in the perspective of the patient's 'lived experience' in nursing care (McKee 1991); and in the value of narrative in medical ethics education (Campbell & Higgs 1982).

The essence of the patient's experience of illness is incapacity, an inability – through pain, distress, paralysis and so on – to do the things one can usually do. It is this incapacity which, as the philosopher Stephen Toulmin (1980) has argued, actually makes us *patients* as distinct from agents. This has some important consequences for theory: it is reflected in the central place of autonomy in health care ethics, for instance; and in the importance of 'empowerment' as a guiding principle in several areas of health care, such as mental handicap (Pearson 1991) and in nurse education (Ersser & Tutton 1991). It has also been the basis for new and more powerful ways of analysing and understanding the sometimes bizarre features of patients' experiences of *mental* illness, in particular delusions and hallucinations (Fulford 1989, ch. 10).

The positive themes of the patient power movement are twinned with two negative themes. The theme of value is twinned with an antifact theme (Alderson 1990). This is because facts and values are often seen as being in conflict. Hence, given that values are important in medicine, it is felt that facts, and with them scientific theories, must be somehow *un*important.

The second positive theme – that of the patient's experience of illness – is twinned with an anti-disease theory theme. Disease theory is built on scientifically derived facts which become no-go areas for anyone who is not an 'expert' (Alderson 1990). Hence the very possibility of patient power is perceived as being dependent on undermining the place of disease theory in medicine, and with it 'the doctor' as an expert on medical science. Science, according to this view, dehumanises the patient, treating her as an object rather than a person, as a machine rather than a moral agent with values and expectations of her own.

The two negative themes in the patient power movement are broadly identifiable with a picture of medicine which has become known as the medical model.

The medical model

The term medical model has been used with a variety of meanings (Macklin 1973). It is the core features of the model, however, which correspond directly with the negative themes of the patient power movement. Thus, according to the medical model, medicine is, essentially, a factual discipline based on scientific knowledge of bodily and mental functioning, knowledge which forms the basis for a set of disease theories to which doctors, in particular, are experts.

Put baldly, this is too extreme a model of course. Nowadays, most health care professionals, most doctors indeed, recognize that there is more to medicine merely than facts, disease theories, and scientific knowledge of abnormal functioning. They recognize, corresponding with the first of the two positive themes of the patient power movement, the importance of ethics and law; and they recognize, corresponding with the second theme, the importance of better understanding of the patient's actual experience of illness, to the extent at least that this is the basis of the good communication skills which, above all, patients find to be lacking (Chapter 14). But these non-specific elements of health care are, nonetheless, according to the medical model, optional extras, fringe benefits to the central scientific agenda of medicine (Boorse 1975). This is sometimes denied by bioethicists (Gillon 1986). Yet it is evident, for example, in the still hierarchical organization of medical practice around doctors, in the almost exclusively scientific basis of medical training, and in the priorities of medical research funding.

This modified medical model – in which the patient's values and experiences are now recognized but remain of only marginal importance – could be a correct picture of medicine. After all, science, which is still central in this model, has been crucial to medical advance. Moreover, if this *is* a correct picture, it would certainly explain why a patient power movement has sprung up. For the medical model suggests that doctors should be concerned at least *centrally* with facts and disease theories, and at best only *peripherally* with the patient's values and experiences of illness. Yet it is the latter which, as the positive themes of the patient power movement show, are at the centre of our concerns as patients. So if this modified medical model is a correct picture of medicine, there is a built-in mismatch between patients and doctors.

But *is* it a correct picture? In the next section this question will be examined, taking psychiatry as a case in point.

Psychiatry and the medical model

Psychiatry is an area in which issues of patient power are particularly acute. In general medicine the problem has been a degree of paternalism which at times has become oppressive and overbearing (Weatherall 1994). But the circumstances are rare indeed in which a doctor can treat a physically ill patient directly against his or her clearly expressed wishes. In psychiatry, on the other hand, involuntary (or compulsory) treatment is an everyday occurrence, the psychiatrist's powers in this respect carrying the force of law (Wing 1978).

The belief that involuntary treatment of psychiatric patients is sometimes justified is widely held (Fulford 1991). It depends on the idea that at least some mentally ill people are not responsible for their actions. Yet precisely *why* this should be so, and hence exactly *which* patients are appropriately treated in this way, remains highly controversial (Szasz 1963). Moreover the widespread abuses of psychiatric patients, institutionalized in the former USSR for instance (Bloch & Chodoff 1977), and probably also in other countries (Fulford *et al.* 1993), shows the extent to which involuntary psychiatric treatment is ethically suspect. There are thus important moral dilemmas here, focusing directly on the power relationships between doctor and patient.

The moral dilemmas raised by involuntary psychiatric treatment have led to an active debate over many years about the very status of psychiatry as a properly medical discipline. Sometimes called the 'debate about mental illness', this has been pursued between those, like Szasz (1960), who argue that mental illness is really a moral concept, and others, like Kendell (1975), who argue that it is a genuinely medical concept. The issues here have generated a large literature (Clare 1979). What has not been widely recognized, however, is that, remarkably, *both* sides in this debate share a conventional medical model of the medical concepts.

There are in fact a whole series of points at which the two sides in the debate about mental illness coincide (Fulford 1989, ch. 1). The key point for us here, though, is this: both sides have assumed that mental illness is a more problematic concept than physical illness because it is more *value-laden*. Now, mental illness certainly is more value-laden; mental illness, for example, connects with moral concepts (e.g. hysteria connects with malingering, alcoholism with drunkenness, psychopathy with delinquency). Even in modern supposedly scientific classifications, a number of mental disorders are still defined by reference to social-evaluative norms (in the American DSM-IV – Diagnostic and Statistical Manual, 4th edn – for example, sexual deviation, or paraphilia, is defined as behaviour which is unacceptable to a majority in the culture from which the patient comes (APA 1994).

Both sides in the debate about mental illness, then, implicitly adopting a conventional fact-centred medical model, have focused on the more value-laden nature of mental illness. They have interpreted this quite differently, however. Szasz (1960) has taken the value-laden nature of mental illness to show that it is not a properly 'scientific' concept, based on factual norms of bodily structure and functioning, and hence that it is a myth. Kendell (1975) on the other hand, relying on the same fact-based medical model, argues that the evaluative connotations of mental illness are merely superficial. Mental illness, he claims, is fully capable of being defined in a straightforwardly empirical way, of being tidied up to make it into a purely scientific (and hence properly medical) concept just like physical illness.

This could be a useful debate. Szasz's insistence on the value-laden nature of mental illnesses could point to the importance of the patient's values and experience of illness; while Kendell's emphasis on the scientific aspects of mental illness could help to ensure that we retain an appropriately scientific basis for treating mental disorders. In other words, the debate could have offered a balance. In fact, though, it has been highly divisive, with pro- and anti-psychiatrists taking up ever more extreme positions, and patients (especially with care in the community (CSAG 1995)) falling between them.

We need a different model – one which avoids the limitations of the medical model. Philosophical analysis, as we noted earlier, is directly concerned with models, with the frameworks of concepts and ideas by which we structure our experience. Philosophical analysis thus offers one method, one set of skills, by which we might come to a better model. In the case of the medical model, moreover, and the debate about mental illness, there are some helpful philosophical ideas on value terms already available to us in the work of Urmson (1950), Hare (1963) and others. It is to these ideas that we turn in the next section.

A model for patient-centred care

The starting point for the philosophical work just mentioned is the observation that value terms, although indeed often obviously value laden, can sometimes look just like factual terms. This is true not only of the terms illness and disease, but even of what we might call general purpose value terms like good and bad. To take a non-medical example, if you are buying apples from the grocer and ask for 'a pound of good eating apples, please', you mean a pound of apples which are sweet, clean-skinned and so on. The meaning of good in this context is thus fact-laden (it conveys sweet, clean-skinned, etc.) rather than value-laden. It is easy to think of other examples of such fact-laden uses of good and bad from everyday experience. But in other situations good is more obviously value-laden, for example in arguments about whether a play is a good play or a picture a good picture.

This observation, that *all* value terms, even good and bad, can sometimes be value-laden is highly relevant to the debate about mental illness. The medical model, as we have seen, has led to a polarization of the debate between those, like Szasz, who take the value-laden nature of mental illness to show that it is not a medical but a moral concept; and those, like Kendell, who believe that mental illness has to be purged of its value-laden nature in order to make it into a properly medical concept. But if illness is a *value* term, and thus has the same properties as good, there is no reason at all why it should not sometimes be fact-laden, as in physical illness, and sometimes value-laden, as in mental illness; that is to say, *physical* illness (fact-laden) and *mental* illness (value-laden), could be, in this respect, just like good *apple* (fact-laden) and good *picture* (value-laden).

This gives a different, and reconciling, alternative to the traditional polarized debate about mental illness. Instead of arguing (with Szasz) that because mental illness is value-laden it is not illness, or (with

Kendell) that mental illness has to be purged of its value-laden nature, this account suggests that *both* concepts are equally valid species of illness. Mental illness (value-laden) and physical illness (fact-laden) are both equally valid species of the value term illness, just as good picture (value-laden) and good apple (fact-laden) are equally valid species of the value term good.

To see the practical consequences of this, however, we need to look at just why it is that value terms have this chameleon-like quality of appearing sometimes in fact-laden and sometimes in value-laden forms. There are a number of reasons for this, again explored by philosophers such as Hare (1963) and Urmson (1950). Perhaps the most important, however, and certainly the most practically significant, is that this property of value terms reflects the extent to which people are in agreement or disagreement on questions of value.

The core idea here is again quite straightforward. I will first state the point and then give an example. It is also illustrated by Fig. 1.1.

The point is that when we use a value term (such as good or illness) we draw on certain *factual* criteria for the value judgement we are expressing. If there is general agreement on these factual criteria, they can become stuck by association to the meaning of the value term in question; but if there is wide disagreement, there is no stable factual meaning to become stuck in this way.

Thus, returning to our example of apples and pictures, more or less everyone agrees that clean-skinned, sweet, etc. apples are good apples. This is not always true (good cider apples are rotten!), but because it is usually true, clean-skinned, sweet, etc. have become stable factual criteria for the value judgement 'good apple'. 'Good' used of apples has thus come to be fact-laden, the factual meaning clean-skinned, sweet etc. having become stuck to it by association. Conversely, though, where people by and large agree over what makes a good apple, they disagree profoundly over what makes a good picture. Hence there is no stable factual meaning to become stuck by association to the value judgement 'good picture'. 'Good' used of pictures thus remains a clearly value-laden term.

Granted, therefore, that illness is a value term, there is a clear possibility that similar factors could be behind the difference between mental illness (value-laden) and physical illness (fact-laden). I have set this out in detail elsewhere (Fulford, 1989). But we can see, at least, that this possibility is consistent with the fact that people differ relatively widely over their value judgements of typical symptoms of mental illness, like anxiety, while they are largely in agreement over their value judgements of typical symptoms of physical illness, like pain.

In the case of anxiety, there is nothing odd about one person enjoying, say, hang-gliding while another dislikes it. This is not a matter of one person feeling anxious while the other does not; it is simply that one enjoys the thrill of fear (she values it positively) while the other does not (she values it negatively). So people differ over their value judgements of anxiety. With pain, by contrast, there is a marked

Apples   *Pictures*

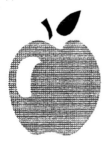   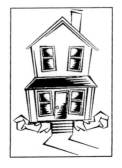

Agreement   *Disagreement*
over what makes a good apple   over what makes a good picture
(sweet, clean-skinned, etc.)   (????)

Hence   *Hence*
the term 'good apple' has acquired   the meaning of 'good picture' has
the factual meaning 'sweet, clean   acquired no consistent factual
skinned, etc.'   meaning

Fig. 1.1 Why value terms (like 'good') can sometimes look like factual terms.

Most people agree that a good apple is one which is sweet, clean-skinned, etc. It is for this reason that the term 'good apple', although expressing a value judgement, conveys the *factual* meaning 'sweet, clean-skinned, etc'. But there is no corresponding agreement about what makes a good picture. Hence, in the absence of a stable factual meaning, the term 'good picture' remains clearly *value* laden. It is for similar reasons that in health care, the term 'physical illness' is relatively fact-laden and 'mental illness' relatively value-laden (see also text).

convergence of values. For almost everyone, pain is at best a necessary evil. Indeed, there would be something distinctly odd about someone who seeks out the pain-equivalent of hang-gliding. As Fig. 1.1 illustrates, then, anxiety is in this respect like pictures, pain like apples. And for this reason alone, the concept of mental illness (made up of phenomena like anxiety) will be more value-laden, while that of physical illness (made up of phenomena like pain) will be more fact-laden.

This conclusion, drawn as it is from philosophical moral theory, gives us a quite different model of health care. As we saw earlier, the medical model, even in its modified form, allows values and the patient's experience to come in only at the margins. Arguments of the kind just outlined show, on the contrary, that values run right through health care (Fulford 1989). For what they show is that even such scientific sounding (or fact-laden) terms as illness and disease are, in reality, value terms. And what this in turn shows is that values, and with them the patient's experiences of illness, are integral, not peripheral, in health care.

Instead of the fact-based medical model, then, we have a more balanced fact + value model. This has important theoretical implications, for diagnosis as well as treatment (Fulford 1993), for secondary as well as primary care (Mayou & Hawton 1986; Wartman *et al.* 1983), and indeed for physical medicine generally as well as psychiatry (Fulford 1989; Hope & Fulford 1993; Kent Kwoh *et al.* 1992). It is, though, the practical implications of a balanced model which show it to be a model for patient-centred health care.

Practical implications of a balanced model of health care

In a balanced model, the clinical and basic sciences are no less important than in the traditional medical model. This first practical point emerges particularly strongly from the philosophical approach just outlined. As noted earlier, where those in the patient power movement have argued for the importance of values in health care, this has generally been in contradistinction to science.

The approach from philosophical moral theory, on the other hand, shows the central importance of values but without in any way undermining the importance of facts. This is partly because, as we have just seen, facts and values are recognized to be woven together in health care. But it is also, and more specifically, because the approach emphasizes the significance of the factual criteria for value judgements. Without these, values have no content, no concrete application. Hence this approach, far from undermining facts, actually demands that we do everything we can – by accurate clinical observation (including listening carefully to the patient) and by whatever scientific tests are appropriate – to provide the securest possible factual basis for the value judgements which, according to this model, permeate all aspects of health care.

A second practical point is the converse of this: although not undermining science, a balanced model adds to it what we can call broadly the human aspects of health care. This is illustrated by Fig. 1.2. Where the medical model treats the patient's values and experience of illness as marginal – giving facts and disease theory central place – a balanced model puts values and facts, illness experience and disease theory, on an equal footing. This is not, as in political and social theory, merely an ideal, something towards which we should strive because it is good. It is, rather, a logical necessity. This is the most compelling of all necessities, for it is a necessity which is driven by the very meanings of the terms (such as health, illness and disease) by which the discipline itself is defined.

One important practical consequence of this (logically necessary) equality is that it helps to balance the power relationship between patients and professionals without the need for being anti-science. To

The medical model

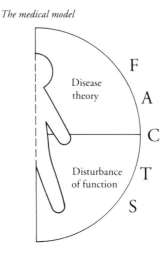

A balanced model

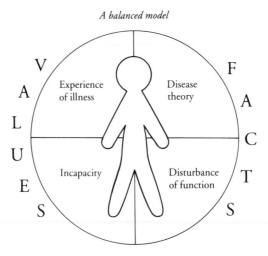

Fig. 1.2 From the medical model to a balanced model of health care.

The facts and scientific disease concepts emphasized in the traditional medical model represent only one half of the conceptual structure of health care. A 'full-field' or balanced model, on the other hand, recognizes the equal importance of values and the patients' experiences of illness. It is a model of this kind which is the basis for genuinely patient-centred care (see also text).

the extent that the medical model has claimed an exclusive or even central place for science in medicine, the patient power movement has been properly directed against it. But there is no corresponding requirement for an anti-science theme if the new model described here, a balanced model, is correct. For in this model the patient's values necessarily stand alongside and equal to the scientific facts. The power of the patient is thus automatically increased.

Balancing the power relationship between doctor and patient is important, not least, ethically, for much unethical practice arises from an imbalance of power in the relationship between patient and professional (Fulford *et al.* 1993). But a balanced model also balances the power relationships between different health care disciplines. Psychiatry, nursing, general practice, and other areas of primary care, are all regarded, in the medical model, as Cinderella disciplines. Being more value-laden, they are considered less 'scientific'. In consequence they have had less influence, resourcing and prestige, and their patients have suffered accordingly.

A balanced model, on the contrary, shows that these disciplines, precisely because they are more overtly value-laden, are not *less* scientific, but, as it were, *more* humanistic. They incorporate in principle all the scientific challenges of technological medicine, but ethical and conceptual challenges as well, challenges which arise, at root, from the necessity (the logical necessity) in these disciplines for dealing with patients as *people*. It is for this reason, indeed, that in both research and health care education, nursing has taken a particular lead in developing methods which are well tuned to the experiential aspects of health care (see for example Chapters 4 and 12).

This is all very well, some may say, but if value judgements are involved in every aspect of health care – even in technical aspects of diagnosis – does it not follow that anything goes? Surely we need the objective facts of science to pin down health care practice?

The answers to these questions will lead to two further important practical points, the first about diagnosis, the second about the multidisciplinary team. The answer to the first question is no, it does not follow that anything goes. Law, for instance, is heavily value-laden, more obviously so even than health care; but we would not say that in law anything goes. Law is a human creation, certainly, rather than a product of scientific research into the nature of things, but human beings are at least to a degree consistent in their judgements of right and wrong, and law, correspondingly, is to a degree consistent. The same is true even for taste, as in our earlier example of apples. The same is true, then, for health; so long as human beings are to a degree consistent in their judgements of health and disease, a balanced model of health care will to the same degree generate clear and consistent diagnostic practices (Fulford 1993).

This is especially important in mental health, where sociological critical theory has often been concerned to show that, because psychiatric diagnosis is value-laden, the whole business of diagnosis in psychiatry should be jettisoned (Coulter 1973). Diagnosis, as this tradition emphasizes, can certainly be dehumanizing; this corresponds with an over-emphasis on the right half of the model illustrated in Fig. 1.2 – the domain of the old medical model.

But to reject diagnosis altogether is to throw out the baby with the bathwater. There is a renewed danger of this happening with the move to community care: a wholesale rejection of diagnostic categories by some community workers, resulting in the neglect of just those patients, such as those with chronic schizophrenia, who are in most need of help (CSAG 1995).

There is nothing patient-centred, then, about giving up diagnosis and all the resources of science which go with it. Uses of diagnosis which ignore its human context are, certainly, *mis*uses of diagnosis. Such misuses include labelling individual patients as diseases ('the CA lung in bed 3 . . .'), or denying the reality of the patient's experience of illness merely because diagnostic tests are negative ('there's nothing medically [sic] wrong with you . . .'); or simply pressing on with intrusive diagnostic procedures without regard to the wishes of patients and relatives. But it is equally wrong to go the other way, to neglect altogether the sound knowledge base for decision making in health care represented by diagnostic categories.

The other side to this coin, though, and this will lead to my last practical point (about the multidisciplinary team), is that while a balanced model does not lead to anarchy, to 'anything goes', it does show that there are definite and proper limits to diagnostic agreement. If diagnosis were entirely (rather than just to an important extent) based on facts, diagnostic agreement would be limited only by the limitations of our existing clinical sciences. But a balanced model shows that diagnosis, especially in psychiatry and other areas of primary care, will *always* be to a degree uncertain, whatever progress is made in science.

This follows from the fact noted earlier that people often differ from one another on matters of value. Most people, as we saw, agree in their value judgements of things like apples and pains, but among the things over which people may disagree are mental symptoms such as anxiety. We found mental symptoms to be, in this respect, like pictures rather than apples. And the point is that this is *not something which science can, or indeed should, change*. It is a feature, an important and legitimate feature, of our *very nature as human beings*. Our similar evaluations of pains (and apples), our dissimilar evaluations of anxiety (and pictures), are not the results of scientific discovery. They are givens of our psychology. Hence while a balanced model is not a recipe for anarchy, it does show that in psychological medicine (and indeed in primary care generally, Fulford 1989, ch. 11), issues of value will always be important in diagnosis, whatever developments take place in science, so long as we are human beings with human natures.

According to a balanced model, then, patients' values can never be supplanted by scientific advance. Again, this is not a matter of political or moral ideals; it is, simply, but far more compellingly, a matter of logic. Patients' values are built into the very meanings of terms like health, illness and disease. A model of health care, therefore, which fails to recognize this is, literally, meaningless.

What should happen in cases where values conflict, then? For scientific questions can, in principle, be settled by reference to 'the facts'. But with questions of value, while issues of relevant fact may be important, there are by definition no objective tests.

It is here that the last practical point, about the multidisciplinary team, finally comes in. In cases where values conflict, it would be easy to say that the patient's express wishes should prevail. This would be one way of understanding the patient-power movement, and certainly there are many situations in which a more sensitive attention to the patient's wishes would result in better care. But what about children, or the mentally handicapped, the confused, the frightened, the mentally ill? Clearly, while avoiding the abuses of an excessively paternalistic use of professional power, it would be wrong to say that in each and every case, the patient's express wishes should prevail. This would not be genuinely patient-centred *care*. It would be a consumer model of health, in which the supplier of goods has merely to flatter the customer with what she wants. But the health care professional has an obligation to *care* (Fulford 1994b).

What is needed is thus a balance of values and it is this which is supplied by the multidisciplinary team. For history shows that in physical medicine as well as in psychiatry, abusive practices are most likely to arise where the values of any one professional group, or even of one person, are allowed to become dominant. This was clearly so with the abuse of psychiatric patients in the former USSR for example (Fulford *et al.* 1993). And as Doyal argues in this book, with cultural differences mainly in mind (Chapter 13), abusive practices may, similarly, arise through an unbalanced exercise even of patients' values. A key role of the multidisciplinary team, then, is to provide a balance of evaluative considerations within which health care decisions can be made, neither automatically acceding to the patient's wishes, nor subordinating the patient's wishes to the interests of one or other professional power group.

Conclusions

What, then, is patient-centred health care? In this chapter this question has been explored by contrasting the concerns of the patient power movement with those of the traditional scientific medical model. This has led to a new model, a fact + value model, which provides a balanced framework for patient-centred care.

The key feature of this model is that it recognizes and makes explicit the way in which values as well as facts are woven together into the very fabric of every aspect of health care. This feature of the model has been derived, not empirically, but from a (logical) property which the terms illness and disease share with all other value terms.

This property, abstract as it is, has generated a series of practical balances which together form a basis for genuinely patient-centred care, a balance between science and the humanities, between disease categories and patients' experiences of illness, between technological medicine and primary care, and, most important of all, a balance between the patient's wishes (emphasized in a patient-power model) and the professional's understanding of their needs (emphasized in the traditional medical model). The trick, though, is to strike these balances appropriately. It is here, as we have just seen, that the multidisciplinary team has an essential role to play.

It is the multidisciplinary team, broadly conceived, which is represented by the diverse contributions to this book. Each chapter illustrates, primarily through the work of its author, a contribution to patient-centred health care. The model of patient-centredness implied by all this is not an easy one to achieve. It is easy to gesture towards team work while reserving a secret priority for one's own profession. There are new roles here for education and training (Chapter 11). There are new roles for audit and evaluation (Chapter 15). But at the end of the day, a balanced model of health care offers no privileged professional centre for the doctor, for the nurse, or for any other professional – or indeed for the patient.

Teams do need leaders, of course. But there is no reason why, in the diversity of modern health care, team leaders should be drawn from any one profession. Horses must, rather, be matched to courses. It is through a dynamic, open approach, therefore, reflective and renewing, in which the full resources of the multidisciplinary team can be deployed, responsive but not subordinate to patients' wishes, that genuinely patient-centred care will be achieved.

Reading Guide

Useful introductions to philosophical work in health care from nursing and primary care perspectives include Chinn and Kramer (1991), Kitson (1993) and Wilson (1963). The background theory to this chapter is set out in detail in my *Moral Theory and Medical Practice* (Fulford 1989, reprinted in paperback 1995). Work on the concept of health (as distinct from illness and disease) includes Nordenfelt's *On the Nature of Health: An Action-Theoretic Approach* (Nordenfelt 1987) and David Seedhouse's *Health: the Foundations of Achievement* (Seedhouse 1986).

Clare (1979) provides a most helpful introduction to the debate about mental illness; and Caplan *et al.*'s *Concepts of Health and Disease* (Caplan *et al.* 1981) offers a valuable collection of primary papers. The use of philosophical analysis in health care is described in more detail in Fulford 1990. This approach is complementary to qualitative methods for the study of patients' lived experiences (see, for example, Chapters 4 and 12 of this book). Journals focusing primarily on the philosophy of health care, as distinct from ethics, include *The Journal of Medicine and Philosophy*, *Theoretical Medicine* and *PPP – Philosophy, Psychiatry and Psychology*.

References

Agich, G.J. (1983) Disease and value: a rejection of the value-neutrality thesis. *Theoretical Medicine*, **4**, 27–41.

Alderson, P. (1990) *Choosing for Children; Parents' Consent to Surgery.* Oxford University Press, Oxford.

APA (1994) *Diagnostic and Statistical Manual of Mental Disorders,* 4th edn. American Psychiatric Association, Washington.

Beauchamp, T.L. & Childress, J.F. (1989) *Principles of Biomedical Ethics.* Oxford University Press, Oxford.

Bloch, S. & Chodoff, P. (1977) *Russia's Political Hospitals.* Camelot, Southampton.

Boorse, C. (1975) On the distinction between disease and illness. *Philosophy and Public Affairs,* **5**, 61–84.

Campbell, A.V. & Higgs, R. (1982) *In that Case: Medical Ethics in Everyday Practice.* Darton, Longman and Todd, London.

Caplan, A.L., Engelhardt, T. & McCartney, J.J. (eds) (1981) *Concepts of Health and Disease: Interdisciplinary Perspectives.* Addison-Wesley, Reading, Massachusetts.

Chinn, P.L. & Kramer, M.K. (1991) *Theory and nursing: a systematic approach,* 3rd edn. Mosby Year Book, St Louis.

Clare, A. (1979) The disease concept in psychiatry. In: *Essentials of Postgraduate Psychiatry* (eds P. Hill, R. Murray & A. Thorley. Grune & Stratton, New York.

Coulter, J. (1973) *Approaches to Insanity: a Philosophical and Sociological Study.* Martin Robertson, London.

CSAG (1995) *Report of the Clinical Standards Advisory Group on Schizophrenia (volume 1).* HMSO, London.

Ersser, S.J. & Tutton, E. (1991) Primary nursing – a second look. In: *Primary Nursing in Perspective* (eds S.J. Ersser & E. Tutton). Scutari Press, London.

Fulford, K.W.M. (1989, reprinted 1995) *Moral Theory and Medical Practice.* Cambridge University Press, Cambridge.

Fulford, K.W.M. (1990) Philosophy and medicine: The Oxford connection. *British Journal of Psychiatry,* **157**, 111–15.

Fulford, K.W.M. (1991) The concept of disease. In: *Psychiatric ethics,* 2nd edn (eds S. Bloch & P. Chodoff). Oxford University Press, Oxford.

Fulford, K.W.M. (1993) Value, action, mental illness and the law. In: *Criminal Law: Action, Value and Structure* (eds S. Shute, J. Gardner & J. Horden). Oxford University Press, Oxford.

Fulford, K.W.M. (1994a) Closet logics: hidden conceptual elements in the DSM and ICD classifications of mental disorders. In: *Philosophical Perspectives on Psychiatric Diagnostic Classification* (eds J.Z. Sadler, M. Schwartz & O. Wiggins). The Johns Hopkins University Press, Baltimore.

Fulford, K.W.M. (1994b) Medical education: knowledge and know-how. In: *Ethics and the Professions* (ed. R. Chadwick). Avebury, Aldershot.

Fulford, K.W.M., Smirnoff, A.Y.U. & Snow, E. (1993) Concepts of disease and the abuse of psychiatry in the USSR. *British Journal of Psychiatry,* **162**, 801–10.

Gillon, R. (1986) *Philosophical Medical Ethics.* Wiley, Chichester.

Hare, R.M. (1963) Descriptivism *Proceedings of the British Academy,* **49**, 115–34. Reprinted in *Essays on the Moral Concepts* (1972, R.M. Hare). Macmillan, London.

Hope, R.A. & Fulford, K.W.M. (1993) Medical education: patients, principles and practice skills. In: *Principles of Health Care Ethics* (ed. R. Gillon). Wiley, Chichester.

Kendell, R.E. (1975) The concept of disease and its implications for psychiatry. *British Journal of Psychiatry,* **127**, 305–15.

Kent Kwoh, C., O'Connor, G.T., Regan-Smith, G., Olmstead, E.M., Brown, L.A., Burnett, J.B., Hochman, R.F., King, K. & Magon, G.J. (1992) Concordance between clinician and patient assessment of physical and mental health status. *Journal of Rheumatology*, **19**, 1031–7.

Kitson, A. (1993) Formalising concepts related to nursing and caring. In: *Nursing: Art and Science* (ed. A. Kitson). Chapman & Hall, London.

Lockyer, D. (1981) *Symptoms and illness: the cognitive organization of disorder.* Tavistock, London and New York.

Macklin, R. (1973) The medical model in psychoanalysis and psychotherapy. *Comprehensive Psychiatry*, **14**, 49–69.

Mayou, R. & Hawton, K. (1986) Psychiatric disorder in the general hospital. *British Journal of Psychiatry*, **149**, 172–90.

McKee, C. (1991) Breaking the mould: a humanistic approach to nursing practice. In: Nursing as Therapy (eds R. McMahon & A. Pearson). Chapman & Hall, London.

Nordenfelt, L. (1987, reprinted 1995) *On the Nature of Health: an Action–Theoretic Approach.* D. Reidel, Dordrecht, Holland.

Pearson, A. (1991) Taking up the challenge: the future for therapeutic nursing. In: *Nursing as Therapy* (eds R. McMahon & A. Pearson). Chapman & Hall, London.

Reich, W. (1991) Psychiatric diagnosis as an ethical problem. In: *Psychiatric Ethics*, 2nd ed (S. Bloch & P. Chodoff), pp. 101–35. Oxford University Press, Oxford.

Rogers, A., Pilgrim, D. & Lacey, R. (1993) *Experiencing Psychiatry: Users' Views of Services.* Macmillan, London.

Sedgwick, P. (1973) Illness – mental and otherwise. *The Hastings Center Studies* **I** (3), 19–40. Institute of Society, Ethics and the Life Sciences, Hastings-on-Hudson, New York.

Seedhouse, D.F. (1986) *Health: the Foundations for Achievement.* Wiley, Chichester.

Szasz, T.S. (1960) The myth of mental illness. *American Psychologist*, **15**, 113–18.

Szasz, T.S. (1963) *Law, Liberty and Psychiatry: an Inquiry into the Social Uses of Mental Health Practices.* Macmillan, New York.

Toombs, S. Kay. (1993) *The Meaning of Illness: a Phenomenological Account of the Different Perspectives of Physician and Patient.* Kluwer Academic Publishers, Dordrecht, The Netherlands.

Toulmin, S. (1980) Agent and patient in psychiatry. *International Journal of Law and Psychiatry*, **3**, 267–78.

Urmson, J.O. (1950) On grading. *Mind*, **59**, 145–69.

Wartman, S.A., Morlock, L.L., Malitz, F.E. & Palm, E. (1983) Impact of divergent evaluations by physicians and patients of patients' complaints. *Public Health Reports*, **98**, 141–5.

Weatherall, D.J. (1994) The inhumanity of medicine: time to stop and think (editorial). *British Medical Journal*, **309**, 1971–2.

Wilson, J. (1963) *Thinking with Concepts.* Cambridge University Press, Cambridge.

Wing, J.K. (1978) *Reasoning about Madness.* Oxford University Press, Oxford.

Commentary on Chapter 1

Roger Higgs

Some may doubt whether patient-centredness in health care is as much part of the scenery as this first chapter suggests. A straw poll of people coming into surgeries or the offices of community health councils might indicate that there are still plenty of experiences to be found which suggest the reverse. As one patient (with a sweet tooth) put it to me recently, if the patient is the centre, it's still more of the 'Polo mint' rather than the 'After Eight' approach to health care for consumers. Perhaps what is clear is that most doctors would be ashamed if they were caught riding roughshod over patients' wishes, and the law has begun to underline this too. The important question remains, however, of how useful the concept is in practice, and how much it is or can be part of real modern health care. Is the concept helpful to the man in the street – or the woman on the long stay ward? Our investigation should take the ideas of this book and place them, squarely and we hope fairly, in the context of current everyday clinical decision making, and see if they get results.

Three areas of clinical work present themselves immediately for examination. The first is that of psychiatry, Fulford's own particular area of clinical work. The contribution of the small but articulate group of patients who are themselves survivors of the system of psychiatric treatment has been a very potent challenge, and will be found particularly germane in this context (Campbell 1993). Current work we are conducting may help to unpick this a little further (pers. comm. to Roger Higgs as part of King's College School of Medicine and Open University preparation for Mental Health course, due in 1996). What is clear at present is that we should note that Fulford's concept of the experience of illness contains at least three elements, which in psychiatry may have widely different readings and consequences in practical terms.

One is the experience of illness itself, which for many psychotic patients who recover remains an event desperately demanding an explanation but usually failing to yield one. The second is the experience of treatment, to which so many have testified. The cruelty which unites so much of what has gone on in the past under the heading of treatment of the mad is very striking. That most of it was not effective probably goes without saying. Yet neither its cruelty nor its ineffectiveness have prevented modern doctors and nurses from also exhibiting treatments which may have very unpleasant and sometimes permanent secondary effects, and, compared with physical treatments, often seem unhelpful to patients themselves.

So to the experience of illness is added the experience of treatment, and lastly the experience of being a patient. Most people do not realize how a serious psychiatric label in itself permanently disables; even for those who have or are largely recovered, it may render them beyond employment or deprive them of basic rights in a way which does not happen even to those previously convicted of criminal charges. To be sure, much of this concerns a dialogue within society in general and not within medicine alone; but doctors remain the advisers of society in this regard, and their views are pivotal. We shall be examining this elsewhere, but I remain unsure as to whether Fulford's ideas will be heard soon enough, and so whether they will be quickly effective in forming a dialogue between the two sides in psychiatry.

My second area for examination is general practice. Here the outcome may be different as Fulford elsewhere has pointed out (Fulford 1989). There is a lot of evidence that general practice, working at peak performance, can provide the focus for just the sort of dialogue that Fulford envisages. The contrast between the living body, lived body and lived self, which Pellegrino and Thomasma (1981) have brought to the forefront of debate and which have become central tenets of nursing ethics, may be useful distinctions here too. A consideration of the experience of being alive and the challenge which illness makes to our own understanding of ourselves is central to much work which goes on in general practice.

The search for the meaning of symptoms is not concerned simply with the search for pathology. That it is so often construed this way has created an instant disappointment system for doctors and their patients which in my view underlies much of the discussion about somatisers (Bass 1990), and so-called heartsink patients, and the increase in complaints to the Family Health Service. It is a major criticism of modern medicine that often no other explanation or utility for symptoms is offered than the presence or absence of physical disease. General practice has tried to make progress by, for instance, understanding why people come to their doctors, what sense can be made of complaints and what patients can learn from them, with the help of social scientists, counsellors, and inspired commentators like John Berger (1967). In this enterprise the balance between the biomedical and biographical is often hard to keep. But at the centre of the quest for meaning lies an assessment of values, primarily that of the patient, but in close second that of the doctor, health professional, or the service itself. This interchange can sometimes seem like a dialogue of the deaf; very often it is carried on without explicit reference, going back and forth as non-verbal communication and creating linkages and clashes which the ear alone finds incomprehensible. In medicine this often causes consultations to be dysfunctional, because we have not learnt, as patients or professionals, Fulford's lesson about the importance of the values which each person brings to a clinical encounter.

A simple example presents itself from my general practice. It concerned treatment recommended by a specialist to a man in his sixties who suffered from angina. The treatment was to lower the patient's cholesterol. Taken with a strict diet which the patient had imposed upon himself, it was successful. On two occasions the patient had come to the practice with new pains, first in the chest and then in the abdomen, investigated by members of the practice team without conclusion. The third time, the patient came to me with pain in the arm and neck and he said that he now realized that all the pains had occurred when he followed the instruction leaflet in the packet! The leaflet had suggested the pills be taken at a different time from the instructions given to him by the specialist. But each time the patient had done as the leaflet suggested, he now realized, he had developed pains. He was convinced that following the instructions was the cause of all his pains; and so was I, after he had explained (deferentially) his theory.

We then tried to negotiate the next move, and at this juncture got into a muddle. I suggested he stop the pills; at first I did not realize that he wanted to carry on. My own values suggested that, dreadful as a heart attack might be in process or consequence, living in repeated pain would be worse. The patient took exactly the opposite view. I was slightly ashamed of our previous failure to diagnose and did not want to cause him distress by my treatment; he did not want to die, but perhaps also, in view of our long and close relationship, did not want to let me down by funking the right and necessary treatment. In microcosm, it was a classic clash between the task of saving life and that of preventing suffering, which comes to a more dramatic head in debates elsewhere.

Eventually we had made our values explicit, and could, with the aid of laughter and an investment in an open relationship, reach a conclusion that seemed good. We had moved the debate on values from the subliminal to the audible. It was a small issue, but without airing it might have led to much more major difficulties: to a sudden death, or to repeated dysfunctional consultations, to non compliance to treatment, or to litigation.

Frequently, in analysing such dysfunctional consultations with medical colleagues in educational settings, one sees the doctor on a high horse galloping off to take the high moral ground, quite unaware of how ineffective, offensive or even ridiculous this might be. A striking parable about this was provided in a completely different context. Nicholas Kraemer, expounding on television his production of an opera *Beauty and the Beast* recorded for television from Tuscany, explained that in his interpretation it was impossible for the Beast to be transformed until Beauty could get off her pedestal and become aware of her imperfections. She was so aware of her high moral values that she was in danger of denying them all by her treatment of the Beast. In her change of heart a kiss, the acknowledgement of her 'beastliness', transformed him to his 'beauty'. The unreflective Pharisaism which held her back was very like the attitude of health care professionals, and seems sometimes to prevent the very people whom they are advising from making the necessary moves, particularly lifestyle changes. The price has been raised too high. A recent debate in the British Medical Journal on whether smokers should be denied coronary artery surgery has demonstrated a similar process (BMJ 1993). Substitute overworking for smoking and doctors begin to see the point. Patients may value health less than other things in their lives, or may balance the conflicting values in a different way. If this is not understood, they cannot hear the message which is intended to improve their health.

Where medical activity merges with the ordinary things people do, unexplained values may most frequently wait to ensnare us. The 'natural' transitions of birth and death provide cogent examples. We reported a case where an elderly cricketer, in pain from a gangrenous leg, was advised to have an amputation (Higgs *et al.* 1987). He declared he was a sportsman, valued his legs, and wished to keep them. The surgeon declared he was toxic from the gangrene, and depressed, and would feel better after amputation. He brought in other amputees to persuade the patient, to no avail. He frankly declared the patient would die without amputation. The patient retorted that as a lonely widower, that is just what he would like to happen. A psychiatrist declared the patient's depressed mood to be within normal limits. The surgeon was finally prevented from trying to take the matter to law by the intervention of a GP and a geriatrician. Terminal care was instituted and the patient died peacefully.

Exploration afterwards suggested that both the patient and the surgeon were deeply sincere and well meaning. For the doctor, his task was to save life at all costs; to the patient, losing a leg was too great a cost. He had made sense of his own life and its tragedies by seeing physical integrity as of major importance. He wished to conclude his life by dying his own death; if life deprived him of certain things, he saw no point in it continuing. Glover (1988) has suggested that in our lives we can in some senses create ourselves. McIntyre (1985) has outlined the way in which we may make sense of the choices people make through the narratives they wish to write through their lives. He suggests the key ideas are that the events and choices should be made intelligible, that a person should be accountable for the actions and choices and that they should accord with his personal identity. But the crucial features for us here are the legitimation, if it is still needed, of a subjective view of illness and of the values which inform choices around an illness. Even, or particularly, at the time of death these values may be crucial to health care decisions which are made. As I have argued elsewhere, as death approaches, these personal evaluations become more, not less, important (Higgs 1995).

Thus in the three areas of psychiatry, general practice and terminal care, Fulford's arguments present both possible explanations for behaviour, difficulties and processes in health care, and can be of practical use in solving some of the problems which a more paternalistic approach to health care throws up. The emphasis, however, remains on the subjunctive. It might be useful, but what is required to make it so?

The first requirement, rather than that the concepts be completely understood, is a recognition at least that values are part of the equation, and can be identified, if not always discussed. I imagine that most patients would want to be seen by a doctor who at least respected their ideas and aims, even if they did not share a similar point of view. On the doctor's part, this might appear to imply a type of chameleon morality, but this is not the case. Much has been written about empathic curiosity (Rogers 1951) and the moral need to see things from the patient's point of view (Campbell & Higgs 1982). This does not necessarily mean any abandonment of the doctor's own personal choices or value for herself, but simply a recognition that the patient's evaluations are real, important, and (probably) of prime consideration. The utility of this in practice is that the doctor should find out what the patient's aims and plans are, not as an additional activity when ordinary medical work gets stuck or problematic, but as an intrinsic part of the work itself. If we agree with Fulford that these concepts are part of real medicine – and I hope it will now be clear that I certainly do – reacting to them or making them real as part of medical work is what stands between their being simply interesting ideas and being critical or vital parts of everyday interactions between patient and professional, or between people and the service they require. The reward of such a re-integration of values in the centre of our work is hard to overstate. Suck it and see, perhaps my patient mentioned at the beginning would have said.

References

Bass, C. (ed) (1990) *Somatization: Physical Symptoms and Psychological Illness.* Blackwell, Oxford.

Berger, J. (1967) *A Fortunate Man.* Allen Lane, London.

BMJ (1993) Should smokers be offered coronary bypass surgery? *British Medical Journal*, **306**, 1047–50.

Campbell, A. & Higgs, R. (1982) *In that Case: Medical Ethic in Everyday Practice.* Darton, Longman and Todd, London.

Campbell, P. (1993) Mental Health Services – the user's view. *British Medical Journal*, **306**, 848–50.

Fulford, K.W.M. (1989) *Moral Theory and Medical Practice*, pp. 23–4. Cambridge University Press, Cambridge.

Glover, J.G. (1988) *I: The Philosophy and Psychology of Personal Identity.* Allen Lane, London.

Higgs, R.H. (1995) *The doctor's duties and the process of dying.* Lecture, April, Otago University, New Zealand.

Higgs, R.H., Livesley, B., Rennie, J. & Relatives (1987) Earning his heroin by seeking release while surgeons advise amputation. *Journal of Medical Ethics*, **13**, 43–8.

McIntyre, A. (1985) *After Virtue.* Duckworth, London.

Pellegrino, E.D. & Thomasma, D.C. (1981) *A Philosophical Basis of Medical Practice.* Oxford University Press, New York.

Rogers, C.R. (1951) *Client Centred Therapy.* Constable, London.

2 ◆ Recovering the Covenant Tradition of Patient-Centred Nursing

Ann Bradshaw

It is often assumed that the nurse is a person who stands within a long tradition of dedicated service, a tradition which she inherits and which will be passed on to future generations. This is wisely and well articulated by Jarvis: '... the nurse is ... the guardian of a tradition about the meaning of nursing into which she inducts her charges'. He quotes Martin Buber: '"Education worthy of the name is essentially education of character", and the character of the nurse is as important as the knowledge that she possesses' (Jarvis 1993). Certainly this was the assumed and often unarticulated consensus of nurses in past generations when the nurse's role was above all else to serve the patient, and nursing was by definition patient-centred. But is this still true today? Does the modern nurse see herself as the guardian of a moral tradition into which future generations of nurses are inducted?

My focus is the changing ideology of nursing and the loss of this tradition. I argue that this change is intimately connected to the rejection of the spiritual dimension of care and has resulted in a movement from patient-centred care to nurse-centred practice. It is important to stress at the outset that although much of the actual care performed by individual nurses ignores prevailing ideologies new ideology inevitably feeds through into practice.

The history and tradition of nursing care

Let us begin by examining the tradition about the meaning of nursing. MacIntyre (1985) has pointed to the vital importance of tradition in understanding contemporary thought. This is profoundly true for nursing. Nursing today is a direct result of its inheritance, and importantly, also of the various reactions to this inheritance. But already this poses a problem, for these reactions have involved a revisionist nursing history which is often simplistic, perpetuating inaccurate misunderstandings of a past that it rejects (Bradshaw 1994). Contemporary nursing writers, drawing on Marxist and feminist analyses, have seen in nursing history a concept of care that is a result of capitalist and patriarchal repression (for example Davies 1980; Salvage 1985; Webb 1986b). The idea of the nurse as a woman whose motivation to care for the sick was inspired by the spiritual ideal of a vocation is considered to be arcane, irrelevant and even a damaging myth that needs dispelling.

Yet it is undoubtedly this very motivation of vocation that has been the driving force in those women, and also men, who sought to practise *caritas*. This concept of care as the virtue of charity is seen by MacIntyre as arising from the Christian imperative of *agape*, love, which went beyond the Greek concept of friendship, *philia*. Here then is an initial grounding for patient-centred care: love for one's neighbour inspired and fundamentally rooted in the covenant love of God for humanity. This was the motivating force for the care of the sick and underlay the charitable fruits of religious revivals through the centuries, particularly in the evangelical revival of the late 18th and early 19th centuries (Chadwick, 1971; Harnack 1961; Troeltsch 1931).

This revival occurred at a time when the spiritual basis of care was weakened, or in Weber's (1991) terminology, routinized. The governing principle of free covenant service in the care of the sick was replaced by that of contractual obligation. In such an era of contractual care, delivered by uncommitted paid servants – 'Sarah Gamp' nurses – Nightingale developed her vision and was led to relocate nursing in its classical covenant tradition in which the care of the sick and the prevention of disease were services to God mediated through the character of the nurse. Character for Nightingale was not merely personality, intuition or feelings, but the practical and moral wisdom resulting from following one's true nature in a response to God. The vocation to care demanded a radical and selfless courage that was not mere duty but was the spiritual response of love (Cook 1913; Nightingale 1873).

This was the basis of Nightingale's disagreement with Mrs Bedford Fenwick over the professionalization of nursing. Nightingale was afraid that the route to professionalization would not only undermine this spiritual basis of care by focusing on the technical and medical, but also that as this basis became marginalized the nurse's care would move from unselfconscious service to the patient towards a self-conscious assertiveness concerned primarily with nursing *per se*. It appears that Nightingale's fears were justified. The movement towards professionalization led to nursing becoming dominated by scientism. In the words of Hewa and Hetherington (1990), nurses were to become 'specialists without spirit'.

Articles in British nursing journals as the century progressed expressed the fears of nurses, often hospital matrons, that as the Judeo-Christian spiritual ethic was becoming increasingly marginalized, the care of patients was growing ever more impersonal; for example, Fox 1912 (Matron of the Prince of Wales' Hospital, Tottenham) and Mac-Manus 1956 (Matron of Guy's). This appears to have been unintentional. Bedford Fenwick (1899) herself pointed to the importance of such values, but these were seen as secondary and marginal to the care of the scientific nurse, rather than as the fundamental dynamic of care. Indeed, it was precisely the motive to re-articulate this increasingly hidden but presupposed tradition that motivated Evelyn Pearce (1967, 1969), the major influence on British nursing from the 1930s to the

1960s but now virtually ignored, and Cicely Saunders, the founder of the modern hospice movement (Du Boulay 1984).

A new basis for nursing

The changing and secular ethos in British nursing, which self-consciously from the 1970s onwards sought to redefine itself in the light of what it saw as an increasingly task-orientated 'bio-medical model' dominated by medicine, has involved a rejection of the values which underlay the tradition itself (Pearson & Vaughan 1986). Rather than reviving its original inspiration by looking backwards at its historical roots and heritage so as to take the tradition forward into the future, as Pearce and Saunders sought to do, contemporary British nursing theorists looked to North American nursing. This radical shift was underpinned by nursing's assertive desire for autonomy as a profession and a search for an academic body of distinctive nursing knowledge. This shifted the focus from service to self, from the patient as the centre of nursing, to an inward concentration on the meaning and value of nursing itself.

North American nursing theory was heavily influenced by Dewey's pragmatism in its growth and development as an academic discipline that was university based. An early nursing pioneer, Annie Goodrich, Dean of Yale University School of Nursing, clearly espoused the belief that scientific 'value-free knowledge' was the basis for nursing (1932). The claims of social scientists, such as Glaser and Strauss (1968), were taken up by nursing philosophers Dickoff and James (1968), to begin to build up this body of nursing knowledge. They argued that theory needed to be developed out of practice, and this belief seemed to provide a way forward for nursing now that its objective framework in the principles of natural law had been rejected. Dickoff and James (1970) were clear that there was no such thing as immutable values; values were to be revalued according to whatever worked practically. Thus, in the early decades of the 20th century, North American nursing took an explicitly pragmatist, philosophically-informed path, unlike British nursing which clung, however subconsciously, to its traditional covenant ethic.

Early nursing theories such as those proposed by Orem (1971, 1980, 1985, 1991), Roy (1976, 1984) and Henderson (1966, 1969) predominantly focused on physical care. The nurse was broadly a manipulator of systems. These objectivist theories were criticised in turn by a growing nursing movement, for their mechanistic and controlling nature which undermined not only the humanity of the patient but also that of the nurse. Existential philosophy and psychology were seen to offer nurses a new basis to practise patient-centred care.

Existentialism is broadly a philosophy of personal experience and meaning. Human individualism and subjectivity are the highest authority, the basis for all knowledge. Each person pursues his or her own existential path towards authentic individual being in the world.

For some philosophers (Kierkegaard 1941; Buber 1958) this path was the Judeo-Christian faith, for others, (Sartre 1965; Nietzsche 1954) the path was that of atheism, despair and nihilism; while for yet others (Heidegger 1962) the path was towards a form of mystical quasi-pantheism.

Existentialism has influenced the growth and development of humanistic psychology, represented by for example Allport 1960; Frankl 1964; Maslow 1968, 1970; May 1983; Rogers 1967. Nursing writers have used existential philosophy and psychology to focus on the subjective experiences of the nurse-patient relationship. Travelbee (1971), for example, drawing on Frankl, is primarily concerned with the nurse being with the patient in order to facilitate his or her search for meaning in the face of suffering. This, too, is Paterson and Zderad's (1976) focus; they explicitly draw on Nietzsche to call for a revaluing of values. The concept of a nursing objectivity is repudiated and the nurse is encouraged to develop an intimate subjective relationship with her patient. But there are problems with this view.

Firstly, and importantly, the physical body becomes marginal to care. This is inevitable, for if subjective, experiential knowledge is the highest authority, the value of systematic, analytic and scientific knowledge is eroded and the physical needs of the body become marginal. Secondly, because existentialism is concerned with individualism, the nature of personal relationships and community is necessarily undermined. It is Buber (1958) and Levinas (1991) who have sought to find human authenticity in personal relationships. For Buber it is in the I–Thou relationship, for Levinas it is in the revelation of the Other, but both these positions are dependent on their grounding in the all embracing Thou, the transcendental Other, the covenant God.

Nursing writers do not embrace these implications. Travelbee's conception of relationship opens her to the same criticisms that Buber levelled at Carl Rogers (1990). For Carl Rogers' (1967) non-directive psychotherapeutic approach depends on an equal and mutual relationship between counsellor and client, taken from Buber's (1958) concept of the I–Thou relationship. But, as Buber (1990) argues, the relationship between helper and helped is not an authentic I–Thou relationship. The helped has needs that the helper does not have, he is vulnerable and the relationship is therefore unequal and inevitably open to manipulation by the stronger partner. Rogers' theory is flawed precisely because he has separated Buber's conception from the validating source.

According to Buber's argument, the very concept of the nurse–patient relationship as a self-consciously psychotherapeutic relationship is not authentic. Without covenant grounding it is not a genuine, mutual, person to person meeting, but rather becomes a therapeutic technique which objectifies the patient and results in an I–It rather than an I–Thou relationship. Furthermore it fails to acknowledge the manipulative power (however unintentional) of the controlling partner, the nurse. Buber's criticism of the Rogerian counselling technique is even more applicable to nursing where, in contrast to psychotherapy, the patient may not even be seeking a psychotherapeutic relationship with the nurse.

But perhaps the most telling problem posed by trying to use existential philosophy as a framework for nursing is revealed by Benner (1984, 1985) and Benner and Wrubel (1989) who are currently very influential in British nursing. Their approach, derived from Heideggerian phenomenology, involves a preoccupation with the nurse's conscious experience of caring as a mode of uncovering nursing meaning.

Yet Heidegger's philosophy is primarily concerned with anxiety in the face of being in the world. It is a philosophy overwhelmingly concerned with finding one's place in being and not with human relationships. It is about self-awareness rather than self-giving. Other people are important only in as much as they too, like us, are concerned to find their place in the world. As Levinas (1989) has argued, Heidegger is primarily concerned with the question 'to be or not to be', whereas the real question, in Levinas' view, is that of the primacy of the calling to the ethical relation: the way of love. The individual is not just 'being' but 'being-for-the-other'; he stands in a face to face relation with his neighbour.

We can therefore argue that Heideggerian phenomenology is unable to provide a basis for patient-centred nursing relationships and a concept of care for others. Instead and inevitably, the self-centred nature of an existential philosophical base used for nursing leads to a preoccupation with self-consciousness and self-awareness and hence a nurse-centred perspective.

Nurse-centred nursing

Current nursing ideas, as we have seen, ultimately lead not only to a repudiation of objective theories and systems of nursing as inauthentic, but also, because of an egocentric nature, the focus is the nurse's self development and hence the empowerment of the nurse's self, particularly, and nursing generally. The repudiation of fixed norms means that conceptual and cultural relativism are introduced. Knowledge is merely dependent on individually or culturally sensed meaning.

This has brought us to a situation in nursing in which there is considered to be no universal truth, only opinions and descriptions disclosable through social science research methodologies. But surely opinion and description (even presuming we can elucidate them correctly) cannot offer generalizable prediction and thus direction for nursing care? In the absence of guiding principles, and in the presence of an inherently unequal nurse-patient relationship, how and by whom is such research to be used? To find answers let us look at two advocates of such research processes: Jane Robinson, Professor of Nursing at Nottingham University, and Christine Webb, Professor of Nursing at Manchester University.

Robinson (1993) argues against the use of paradigms as a basis for nursing knowledge. Instead she calls for the meaning and purpose of nursing to be elucidated through concept clarification and a description of the social processes of nursing. She argues that through an 'existential use of models', she has been able to consider the forces that 'trapped' nursing in its 'invisibility' and this has led her to examine issues of power and control. So we see that the use of social science research is not merely for neutral description, but rather, as Robinson (1992) herself makes clear, to break down any notion of a consensus tradition and hence achieve a measure of prediction, authority and control.

How and why this inevitably happens become clearer with Webb, a feminist, in her discussion about the kind of research she advocates for nursing. 'What happens within the research will be strongly influenced by the personal investment which researchers make in the project' (Webb 1992). This contradicts her own assertions made a few sentences earlier, that action research changes power relationships 'from control by researchers to co-operation among all participants'. But it is consistent with her position, demonstrated in one paraphrased quotation from a critical theorist, Brian Fay (1975), that forms the basis of her position and which is repeated at the beginning and end of her text: nurses must 'actively engage in deciding what it is they are and want, and what arrangements must be altered or established to fulfil themselves' (Webb, 1986a).

Webb is employing a neo-Marxist analysis of nursing, and we can argue that her claims rest on a mask of dogmatism, merely another guise for power. This was indeed Foucault's criticism of Fay's influences, the Frankfurt School and Habermas (Merquior 1985). For when human beings are no longer subject to the values of natural law and universal truth they become subject to their own emotivist impulses. MacIntyre's own analysis (1985) agrees: '... arbitrary will and desire (which) sustain the moral masks of modernity ...'.

This was exactly the kind of shift Nietzsche (1954) had anticipated in his parable of *The Madman*. The madman in the market place uses his lamp to search for God, but God is dead and only a madman looks for him. The madman's lamp lies smashed on the floor and over time the effects of this lamp will gradually wear away. Likewise contemporary nurse theorists have rejected their covenant tradition and, in a similar way to Nietzsche's madman, have broken Nightingale's lamp. According to Nietzsche the full implications of this destruction will become clear over time as the influence of the light from the broken lamp wanes and traditional ethics slowly fade.

Nietzsche (like Foucault after him) saw this truth clearly. He claimed liberation from outdated conventional moralities and hence rejected Kantian ethics. If God is dead then everything is permitted, human rationality cannot discover 'the good' for it nowhere exists objectively. And Nietzsche was right, for Kant's moral outlook presupposed traditional moral values derived from his own sheltered Protestant upbringing (Warnock 1964; Williams 1973). He was sitting on a branch that he had cut away from the tree!

This situation mirrors C. S. Lewis's analysis in *The Abolition of Man* (1978). When objective values are removed, what remains is human subjectivity and the power of what Lewis calls the 'Conditioner': 'When all that says "it is good" has been debunked, what says "I want" remains'. For nursing then, the consequences become clear scientifically-based, reductionist nursing theories with the nurse as a manipulator of human systems have given way to explicitly experiential nursing theories with the nurse as existential interpreter and facilitator of the patient's private world. And notably, from both positions, the nurse is in control; whatever the claims to the contrary, this is nurse-centred nursing. It is therefore ironic for Jane Salvage (1992), who describes herself as 'an active participant' in the changing ideology of nursing, to protest at what is an inevitable result of her policy: the empowerment of nurses not patients. But this policy has been no mere academic theory; it has been implemented in patient care.

The fragmentation of nursing

By rejecting the ethical framework of the tradition, and thereby following Nietzsche's wiping away of the horizons, nursing today has lost its organic unity. It no longer holds to a tradition about the meaning of nursing, the very meaning and purpose of nursing is now no longer clear; see for example Clarke & Wheeler 1992; Ersser 1991; Farmer 1993; Forrest 1989; Kitson 1993; Pearson 1988. This fragmentation is having profound implications for nursing, not only in its theories of caring, but inevitably in the building of these theories and in their dissemination into practice.

And here we can see the relevance for British nursing of Davis' five year study of doctrinal conversion among North American nurses in the 1970s. He observed that nurses who arrived at the outset of training with a loose but broadly altruistic Christian-humanitarian vocational conception of care were, during their courses, deliberately conditioned out of such ideals. This occurred because of what Davis calls 'professional rhetoric ... the psychotherapeutic, educationist and social science' (Davis 1975) terminologies and ideologies that were the prevailing influences in forming 'the doctrine of the school' (Davis 1975).

It seems that British nurses are now following in the path of Davis' nurses. But even so we may wonder if the very concept of nursing as care for others still clings on as a vestige of the past. For it is no longer clear why, having revalued nursing values, 'care' should still be a primary moral imperative. Indeed, Nietzsche (1968) himself regarded the support of the sick and weak as indefensible in the light of his call for power and self-assertiveness. Perhaps nursing theorists like Kant implicitly presuppose the Christian ethic of care, even though they explicitly challenge its basis. Using Berkhof's (1979) analogy, they are taking the gospel fruit while destroying the gospel tree. It is to this traditional nursing ethic I will now turn.

The tradition recovered: the covenant theory of care

The patient as a person

The covenant perspective (articulated for example by Barth 1961) understands the human being as both material body and spiritual essence made in the image and likeness of God. The dignity and value of the human being is thus not dependent on subjective judgements of worth, achievement, personal qualities or social position, but in the equality of his or her createdness in covenant love. Each person is of infinite worth whatever his or her personal or physical condition, or even level of mental consciousness. Health then is the strength to be human, to fulfil human created destiny, a fulfilment that can be achieved whatever, and even despite, physical, mental or social frailty or incapacity. This understanding of health therefore goes beyond its utility for social functioning or personal realization, although it encompasses both aspects. Ultimately health as the strength to be human is connected to the acknowledgement of human purpose.

Hence, because of the real and rational nature of creation, the claims of scientific knowledge are recognized as valid and valuable. As Thomas (1971) points out, Judeo-Christian principles laid the groundwork for the discoveries of natural science in the 17th and 18th centuries, by bringing into decline the pagan belief in magic. Disease, suffering and death are, as far as possible, to be prevented and controlled through the application of scientific principles and not passively accepted. The nurse needs rigorous scientific knowledge and competent practical skill for this purpose.

Nevertheless, as Polanyi (1967) has argued, empirically derived knowledge is necessary but not sufficient. Thus while the covenant approach upholds scientific and technical knowledge and recognizes insights into human behaviour and society elucidated from the human and social sciences, it also warns of the limitation of such knowledge. By preserving the personhood of the individual in the face of scientific reductionism and dualism, the covenant perspective questions purely materialistic nursing theories. But, like Polanyi, who also points to the limits of existentialism, the covenant perspective questions existentially-derived nursing theories that marginalize human physical functioning and devalue objective knowledge gained from the natural sciences. The patient is a physiological, social and psychological animal, but he or she is also more than mere nature, for the spiritual dimension of the person is the animation by the breath of life, the image of God within.

The response of care

The grounding of the nursing ethic in a covenant foundation provides for an understanding of care as a free vocational response to the call to love because of the theological origins of such love, whether the nurse knows it or not. It is thus human nature to care for others, and human destiny is fulfilled when the human being makes a free choice to love. As Williams (1978) writes, in vocation:

> 'The adult status of the sick person is retrieved through the fact that any task performed for him is regarded by the nurse as her privilege, for through it she finds the satisfaction and fulfilment of her calling. The sick person's worth is thus restored through an evaluation of him that transcends the normal and more secular definitions of adulthood.'

The basis of care is therefore objectively grounded and professional love, *agape*, not moderated by contractual principles but rather freely given through a covenant understanding, an unconditional self-giving and unselfconscious sharing of the other person's troubles that does not depend on a response or even a recognition. This is illustrated by the parable of the Good Samaritan. My nursing care is for the person who needs me here and now, regardless of his culture, beliefs, attributes or responsibility (see for example McFarlane 1988).

Yet this is no emotional and subjective involvement with the patient as advocated by existential nursing writers. The inherent inequality of the nurse–patient relationship, as we have seen, together with what Campbell (1984) calls its 'dangerous intimacy', means that the nurse's care is in danger of becoming both self-indulgent and a manipulative technique. Campbell's caution rightly calls into question nursing interventions and activities, both verbal and physical, that intrude into the care of the patient and transgress this intimacy, however well-intentioned such activity might be.

But Campbell only reluctantly uses the concept of covenant as opposed to that of contract to describe the caring relationship. This is because he wants to moderate the kind of love given by the professional carer in order to prevent a too intimate involvement with the cared-for. However love is no longer love when it becomes conditional. The objectivity of the professional loving relationship is not maintained by moderating the *quality* of love but rather it is itself moderated through the covenant *nature* of love. This is because the objectivity of *agape* means that it is different (although not entirely distinct) from *eros*, the hunger for self-satisfaction. Love is not merely an arbitrary emotional response, but the ground of human relationality.

Covenant love then does not call for an emotionally intimate relationship between nurse and patient, but neither does it lead to a relationship of emotional distance and impersonal detachment. Rather, objectivity and subjectivity are held together in their foundation and origin; as Buber understood, the equality of the relationship rests in the transcendent all embracing Thou. The caring relationship therefore has an objectivity that enables sometimes painful tasks to be performed, and also allows for the conclusion and separation of the relationship when it is no longer required.

Theorists who base their concept of caring on Buber's I–Thou relationship without reference to his theological principles misunderstand him. Noddings (1984), for example, uses Buber as a basis for her feminine conception of caring, but asserts that theological principles are 'irreconcilable' with her position: 'Human love, human caring, will be quite enough on which to found an ethic.' But how is human love to be defined? For is it not susceptible to the capriciousness of emotions and, as Nietzsche has shown, the self-centred desires of the will to power? We are neither perfect nor perfectible. We have a shadow side of weakness and limitation. Carl Rogers' optimism about the human condition is misplaced, as history undoubtedly shows (May 1990; Niebuhr 1990). We need only look at nursing studies which show that patients can be difficult and hence unpopular with nurses, and nurses can be cold and uncaring (Stannard 1978; Stockwell 1972). This vital issue, so ignored by contemporary nursing theorists, is confronted with realism and hope by the pattern of the covenant tradition of care.

Patient-centred nursing care: the ethic of service

A good nurse is a good person. The quality of the nurse's care depends on such goodness, reflected in the character of the carer, her or his moral wisdom that offers the response of *agape*. This is expressed in the nurse's attitude to everyday nursing activity, in the freedom of the heart within the face to face encounter, in the genuine kindness, warmth, gentleness, conscientiousness, competence, sensitivity and skill with which she washes her patients, cleans away their excreta, promptly responds to their pain or nausea or toilet needs, performs complex technical tasks, explains procedures and listens to their fears. As Pearce (1969) taught, such care is demonstrated even in the gentle adjustment of the pillows that increases comfort and gives reassurance that the nurse is there.

This was not merely the application of skills and techniques but a genuine relationship. It was an essential requirement of this tradition that shared, honest communication was a prerequisite to care. Pearce (1967, 1969) describes the importance of the nurse listening to the patient's needs, answering his questions and informing him carefully about all procedures and activities. Saunders, too, held such honest and genuine communication to be fundamental to hospice philosophy.

It is interesting, therefore, that Salvage (1990) refers to a study in which patients expressed the basic requirement of nursing care as the need for kindness, which as she points out, does not mean that they require a psychotherapeutic relationship with their nurse. Similarly, Morse *et al.* (1992) question the uncritical influence that Rogerian psychotherapeutic concepts and techniques have had in nursing and

call for a re-examination of the currently devalued strategies of compassion and sympathy. Yet these values are personal qualities not
strategies or techniques. They depend on the character of the carer who
inherits and therefore follows in a moral pattern. The reason they are
now devalued is because this moral tradition, of which sympathy and
compassion was the essence, is now deconstructed. And we might also
ask of the hospice movement and palliative care itself, whether the
increasing application of psychosocial techniques to patient care does
not reflect a similar change?

The importance of communication then is not a recent research
discovery, as suggested by for example Bond and Bond (1986), but was
essential to traditional care. Empirical research studies may discover
fragments of the nature of care, splinters of the broken lamp; they are
unable to provide the whole picture because they reject the ethical
framework. The quality of nursing care – its patient-centredness –
arises both historically and theoretically from the moral covenant framework of our tradition; not from an artificial application of techniques, but from genuine, altruistic service. According to Nightingale
(1882): 'The nurse must have simplicity and a single eye to the patient's
good. She must make no demand for reciprocation, for acknowledgement or even perception of her services . . .'.

This covenant approach was often unarticulated but nevertheless it
was lived out. It was an embodied incarnated ethic, not words but
action: a way of care that was taken for granted as the basis for our
nursing tradition. It offers us, even today, a distinctive unity and
wholeness for a pastoral, genuinely patient-centred way of care. It is
fitting to end with Nightingale's (1888) words: 'Rules may become a
dead letter. It is the Spirit of them that "giveth life".'

Reading guide

Bradshaw, A. (1994) *Lighting the Lamp: the Spiritual Dimension of Nursing Care.*
    Scutari Press, London.
Kirschenbaum, H. & Henderson, V. (eds) (1990) *Carl Rogers: Dialogues.* Con-
    stable, London.
McFarlane, J. (1988) Nursing: a paradigm for caring. In *Ethical Issues in Caring*
    (eds G. Fairbairn & S. Fairbairn). Avebury, Aldershot.
MacIntyre, A. (1985) *After Virtue* 2nd edn. Duckworth, London.
Nightingale, F. (1882) Nursing the sick. In *A Dictionary of Medicine*, part II (ed. R.
    Quain). Longmans, Green & Co, London.
Pearce, E. (1969) *Nurse and Patient*, 3rd edn. Faber & Faber, London.

References

Allport, G. (1960) *The Individual and His Religion.* Macmillan, New York.
Barth, K. (1961) *Church Dogmatics* **3** (3). T. & T. Clark, Edinburgh.
Bedford Fenwick (1899) Religious Liberty (editorial). *Nursing Record and Hos-
    pital World,* **xxiii** (604) 345–6.

Benner, P. (1984) *From Novice to Expert*. Addison-Wesley, Menlo Park, California.

Benner, P. (1985) Quality of life: a phenomenological perspective on explanation, prediction and understanding in nursing science. *Advances in Nursing Science*, **8**(1) 1–14.

Benner, P. & Wrubel, J. (1989) *The Primacy of Caring*. Addison-Wesley, Menlo Park, California.

Berkhof, H. (1979) *An Introduction to the Study of the Christian Faith*. Eerdmans, Grand Rapids.

Bond, J. & Bond, S. (1986) *Sociology and Health Care*. Churchill Livingstone, Edinburgh.

Bradshaw, A. (1994) *Lighting the Lamp: the Spiritual Dimension of Nursing Care*. Scutari Press, London.

Buber, M. (1958) *I and Thou*. T. & T. Clark, Edinburgh.

Buber, M. (1990) Chapter 3 in *Dialogues with Carl Rogers* (eds H. Kirschenbaum & V. Henderson). Constable, London.

Campbell, A. (1984) *Moderated Love*. SPCK, London.

Chadwick, O. (1971) *The Victorian Church*, part 1. A. & C. Black, London.

Clarke, J. & Wheeler, S. (1992) A view of the phenomenon of caring in nursing practice. *Journal of Advanced Nursing*, **17**, 1283–90.

Cook, E. (1913) *The Life of Florence Nightingale*. Macmillan, London.

Davies, C. (1980) *Rewriting Nursing History*. Croom Helm, London.

Davis, F. (1975) Professional socialization as subjective experience: the process of doctrinal conversion among student nurses. In *A Sociology of Medical Practice* (eds C. Cox & A. Mead). Collier-Macmillan, London.

Dickoff, J. James, P. (1968) A theory of theories: a position paper. *Nursing Research*, **17**(3), 197–205.

Dickoff, J. & James, P. (1970) Beliefs and values: bases for curriculum design. *Nursing Research*, **19**(5), 415–27.

Du Boulay, S. (1984) *Cicely Saunders*. Hodder & Stoughton, London.

Ersser, S. (1991) A search for the therapeutic dimensions of nurse–patient interaction. In: *Nursing as Therapy* (eds R. McMahon & A. Pearson). Chapman & Hall, London.

Farmer, B. (1993) The use and abuse of power in nursing. *Nursing Standard*, **7**(23), 33–6.

Fay, B. (1975) *Social Theory and Political Practice*. George Allen & Unwin, London.

Forrest, D. (1989) The experience of caring. *Journal of Advanced Nursing*, **14**, 815–23.

Fox, M. (1912) Nursing ethics. *Nursing Times*, **8**(366), 475–8.

Frankl, V. (1964) *Man's Search for Meaning*. Hodder & Stoughton, London.

Glaser, B. & Strauss, A. (1968) *The Discovery of Grounded Theory: Strategies for Qualitative Research*. Weidenfeld and Nicholson, London.

Goodrich, A. (1932) *The Social and Ethical Significance of Nursing*. Macmillan, New York.

Harnack, A. von (1961) *The Mission and Expansion of Christianity in the First Three Centuries*. Harper Torchbooks, New York.

Heidegger, M. (1962) *Being and Time*. SCM Press, London.

Henderson, V. (1966) *The Nature of Nursing*. Collier Macmillan, London.

Henderson, V. (1969) *Basic Principles of Nursing Care*. International Council of Nurses, Geneva.

Hewa, S. & Hetherington, R. (1990) Specialists without spirit: crisis in the nursing profession. *Journal of Medical Ethics*, **16**, 179–84.

Jarvis, P. (1993) *Nursing: a caring relationship. A response to engaging with the whole person as a person.* Paper given at patient-centred health care multi-disciplinary working group, 22–23 April, Green College, Oxford.

Jones, A. (1871) *Memorials* (ed. by her sister). Strahan & Co, London.

Kierkegaard, S. (1941) *Training in Christianity*. Oxford University Press, London.

Kitson, A. (1993) Formalizing concepts related to nursing and caring. In: *Nursing: Art and Science* (ed. A. Kitson). Chapman & Hall, London.

Levinas, E. (1989) *The Levinas Reader* (ed. S. Hand) Blackwell Publishers, Oxford.

Levinas, E. (1991) *Totality and Infinity*. Kluwer Academic Publishers, Dordrecht.

Lewis, C.S. (1978) *The Abolition of Man*. Fount, Glasgow.

McFarlane, J. (1988) Nursing: a paradigm for caring. In: *Ethical Issues in Caring* (eds G. Fairbairn & S. Fairbairn). Avebury, Aldershot.

MacIntyre, A. (1985) *After Virtue*, 2nd edn. Duckworth, London.

MacManus, E. (1956) *Matron of Guy's*. Andrew Melrose, London.

Maslow, A. (1968) *Toward a Psychology of Being*. Von Nostrand Reinhold, New York.

Maslow, A. (1970) *Motivation and Personality*. Harper & Row, New York.

Maslow, A. (1987) *Motivation and Personality*. (revised by R. Frager, J. Fradiman, C. McReynolds & R. Cox). Harper Collins, New York.

May, R. (1983) *The Discovery of Being*. W.W. Morton & Co., New York.

May, R. (1990) Chapter 9 in *Dialogues with Carl Rogers* (eds H. Kirschenbaum & V. Henderson). Constable, London.

Merquior, J. (1985) *Foucault*. Fontana, London.

Morse, J., Anderson, G., Bottorff, J., Yonge, O., O'Brien, B., Solberg, S. & Hunter McIlveen, K. (1992) Exploring empathy: a conceptual fit for nursing practice. *Image: Journal of Nursing Scholarship*, **24** (2), 373–80.

Niebuhr, R. (1990) Chapter 8 in *Dialogues with Carl Rogers* (eds H. Kirschenbaum & V. Henderson). Constable, London.

Nietzsche, F. (1954) *The Portable Nietzsche* (ed. W. Kaufmann). The Viking Press, New York.

Nietzsche, F. (1968) *Twilight of the Idols/The Antichrist*. Penguin, Harmondsworth.

Nightingale, F. (1860) *Suggestions of Thought to the Searchers after Truth among the Artizans of England* (3 vols). Eyre & Spottiswode, London.

Nightingale, F. (1873, 1888) Letters and addresses to the probationer nurses in the 'Nightingale Fund' School at St. Thomas' Hospital, and nurses who were formerly trained there. Original letters and prints for private circulation held by University College, London.

Nightingale, F. (1882) Nursing the sick. In: *A Dictionary of Medicine*, part II (ed. R. Quain). Longmans, Green & Co, London.

Noddings, N. (1984) *Caring: a Feminine Approach to Ethics and Moral Education*. University of California Press, Berkeley.

Orem, D. (1971) *Nursing: Concepts of Practice*, 1st edn. McGraw-Hill, New York.

Orem, D. (1980) *Nursing: Concepts of Practice*, 2nd edn. McGraw-Hill, New York.

Orem, D. (1985) *Nursing: Concepts of Practice*, 3rd edn. McGraw-Hill, New York.

Orem, D. (1991) *Nursing: Concepts of Practice*, 4th edn. Mosby-Year-Book, St Louis.

Paterson, J. & Zderad, L. (1976) *Humanistic nursing*. Wiley, New York.

Pearce, E. (1967) *A General Textbook of Nursing*, 17th edn. Faber & Faber, London.

Pearce, E. (1969) *Nurse and Patient*, 3rd edn. Faber & Faber, London.

Pearson, A. (1988) *Primary Nursing*. Chapman & Hall, London.

Pearson, A. & Vaughan, B. (1986) *Nursing Models for Practice*. Heinemann, London.

Polanyi, M. (1967) *The Tacit Dimension*. Doubleday Anchor, New York.

Robinson, J. (1992) Introduction: beginning the study of nursing policy. In: *Policy Issues in Nursing* (eds J. Robinson, A. Gray & R. Elkan). Open University Press, Milton Keynes.

Robinson, J. (1993) Problems with paradigms in a caring profession. In: *Nursing: Art and Science* (ed. A. Kitson). Chapman & Hall, London.

Rogers, C. (1967) *On Becoming a Person*. Constable, London.

Rogers, C. (1990) *Carl Rogers: Dialogues* (eds H. Kirschenbaum & V. Henderson. Constable, London.

Roy, C. (1976) *Introduction to Nursing: Adaptation Nursing*, 1st edn. Prentice-Hall, New Jersey.

Roy, C. (1984) *Introduction to Nursing: Adaptation Nursing*, 2nd edn. Prentice-Hall, New Jersey.

Salvage, J. (1985) *The Politics of Nursing*. Heinemann, London.

Salvage, J. (1990) The theory and practice of the 'new nursing'. *Nursing Times*, **86** (4), 42–5.

Salvage, J. (1992) The new nursing: empowering patients or empowering nurses? In: *Policy Issues in Nursing* (eds J. Robinson, A. Gray & R. Elkan). Open University Press, Milton Keynes.

Sartre, J-P. (1965) *Existentialism and Humanism*. Methuen, London.

Saunders, C. (1986) The modern hospice. In: *In Quest of the Spiritual Component of Care for the Terminally Ill* (ed. F. Wald). Yale University Press, New Haven.

Stannard, C. (1978) Old folks and dirty work: the social conditions for patient abuse in a nursing home. In: *Readings in the Sociology of Nursing* (eds R. Dingwall & J. McIntosh). Churchill Livingstone, Edinburgh.

Stockwell, F. (1972) *The Unpopular Patient*. Royal College of Nursing, London.

Thomas, K. (1971) *Religion and the Decline of Magic*. Penguin, Harmondsworth.

Titchin, A. (1993) *Engaging with the whole person as a person: professional craft knowledge in patient-centred nursing*. Paper given at patient-centred health care multi-disciplinary working group, 22–23 April, Green College, Oxford.

Travelbee, J. (1971) *Interpersonal Aspects of Nursing*. F.A. Davis, Philadelphia.

Troeltsch, E. (1931) *The Social Teaching of the Christian Churches*, vols 1 & 2. George Allen & Unwin, London.

Walton, J. (1990) *Method in Medicine*. Harveian Oration of the Royal College of Physicians, London.

Warnock, G. (1964) Kant. In: *A Critical History of Western Philosophy* (ed. D. O'Connor). The Free Press of Glencoe, New York.

Webb, C. (1986a) *Women's Health*. Hodder & Stoughton, London.

Webb, C. (1986b) *Feminist Practice in Women's Health Care*. Wiley, Chichester.

Webb, C. (1992) The use of the first person in academic writing: objectivity, language and gatekeeping. *Journal of Advanced Nursing*, **17**, 747–52.

Weber, M. (1991) *Essays in sociology* (eds H. Gerth & C. Wright Mills. Routledge, London.

Williams, B. (1973) *Problems of the Self*. Cambridge University Press, Cambridge.

Williams, K. (1978) Ideologies of nursing: their meanings and implications. In: *Readings in the Sociology of Nursing* (eds R. Dingwall & J. McIntosh).

Commentary on Chapter 2

John Hall

This chapter addresses a wide range of issues, including the Christian concepts of *agape*, and of vocation, underpinning the classic Nightingale 19th century 'lamp' tradition of nursing. The author offers a detailed analysis of the philosophical implications of the Nietzschian, so-called objectivist, subjectivist, and professional-autonomy-driven models of nursing which have developed, largely in North America. She explores the rediscovery of a covenant theory of care, emphasizing the centrality of the patient as person, and the compassionate nature of the nurse–patient relationship.

This response comes from a perspective of a long-standing interest in both the psychology of nursing and of caring (Hall 1990), and in the field of pastoral care, which is the practical expression of religiously-inspired concern for the needy. This chapter forces us to consider the relationship between, on the one hand, caring contrasted both with counsel and with the technical tasks of medical problem-focused communication and medical treatment, and on the other hand nursing care contrasted with informal care, social care and pastoral care.

For most of history most of humanity has not had treatment or cure as an option; care has been the only response on offer to sickness and disability, and mostly by their families or those whom we now term informal carers. There can be little doubt that 'caring' is rooted in the Christian tradition, predating the foundation of what we would now call the nursing profession by several hundred years. That tradition clearly involved men too, as the evidence of the infirmaries of our oldest cathedrals clearly shows, and as shown by the writings of some of the earliest Christian church fathers from the 3rd century, and other writers such as Thomas Aquinas, Calvin and Wesley (Oden 1983).

The boundaries of many of our present academic disciplines were set during the last century, so that the phenomena of care 'slipped between the tight conceptual categories of the social sciences' (Finch & Groves 1983), and have only recently been identified as a focus of attention in its own right. A casualty of this is that care has been discussed largely by two professions – nursing and social work – and has not been actively related to undergirding academic disciplines. A further problem is that as nurses have become more psychologically minded they have become interested in the clinical and counselling psychologies, and their own analyses of nursing care can convey the idea that 'mere' care is second-best – they are at risk of selling their caring birth-right for a mess of psychological pottage.

The development of nursing as a distinct profession took place within that same ferment of social concern and emergent professionalism of the last century. The range of what we are now – differentiated and separate caring and social services – and the accompanying range of discrete professions or semi-professions, emerged from the complex historical network of charity, poor law, and benefit payments which preceded the present welfare state system (Blaxter 1976; Heasman 1962). Kane and Kane (1982) point out that long-term care is 'a perplexing and ill-defined area', characterized by complexity and ambiguity, by potentially overwhelming issues of numbers, and by potentially enormous cost. Downie and Telfer (1980) discuss in detail the background political and ethical issues of utilitarianism, of the welfare state, and of the place of charitable organizations, that confuse thought in this area.

It is a paradox that in these services developing and becoming separated from the ecclesiastical parish system (Halmos 1965), they shared common charismatic leaders – such as Shaftesbury, Rowntree, and Booth, as well as Nightingale – rooted in the Christian tradition, and ideologies permeated by Christian thinking. More generally, therefore, the whole idea of care can be seen as evoking a range of attitudes, coloured by history and Christian ethics and practice, towards the appropriateness of care and of particular caring agents. As Kitwood (1990) has recently pointed out, 'Western moralism is built . . . upon Greek and Judaeo–Christian foundations'.

Accordingly much of the discussion in this chapter, while drawing attention to the philosophical and religious ideas implicit in nursing care and in other forms of care, applies to care by any person in any setting. A theologically informed commentator such as Campbell (1984) uses categories in describing nursing – 'sexual estrangement', 'angel, mother, or body-expert', 'doing to and being with', and 'nursing as skilled companionship' – which could equally well be used to describe informal caring, or much of social care. Standing outside nursing, nursing has still to define carefully what uniquely defines nursing care.

Health care professionals often use the terms spiritual, religious, and theological interchangeably, without realising the different implications of each concept. An emphasis on the spiritual aspects of care focuses on the 'ultimate' meaning ascribed to illness and experience of treatment and healing (which interestingly emerged as an important element of self-described quality of life in Ray Fitzpatrick's presentation, quoting Cella and Tulsky (1990)).

Religious aspects of care often imply attention paid to formal beliefs and religious practices. Neglected areas of concern are theological concepts of care, applying formal theological ideas, such as that of covenant and vocation, explored by Bradshaw in this chapter. There now exists a considerable theological literature on the theology of caring, much of it focusing on the care of people with learning disability, which has a powerful integrative potential in this field (see, for example, Pailin 1992).

A spiritual approach to care has to take account of our view of personhood, of relationships, and of the meaning of our lives. The central Judaeo–Christian concept of people being made in the image of God has powerful implications for our view of personhood, and a positive model of personhood becomes a prerequisite for the maintenance of quality care, as explored by McFadyen (1990). The social sciences have not been the best source for models of personhood, but a leading philosopher of psychology (Shotter 1980) stresses the need for an 'image of man' – and of woman – as an integral part of our everyday attempt to live our daily lives.

To establish general principles from extreme cases is poor logic, but by contrast the example of the long and sad series of committee-of-enquiry reports in psychiatric hospitals illuminates the end-point of the abuse of power in caring relationships (Hugman 1992). At bottom what is frequently found in abusing relationships is a dehumanising view of personhood, so that carers no longer see people with long-term handicaps as truly human.

Care is experienced relationally as a mutual process, in that the cared-for and the carer usually engage in the caring encounter or interaction. It is as important to examine the beliefs, goals, practices and emotions of the carer as of the cared-for. The theological concepts of *agape* and of compassion (Nouwen *et al.* 1982) reciprocally resonate with secular and theological concepts in a way that is mutually enriching.

Perhaps most significantly, experience of sickness and of care will often be significant life events, and often construed within the personal spiritual framework of the individual, as well as within a life events framework. There is thus a benefit to adopting a life journey, or developmental, approach to the person's experience of patienthood and to their health and religious beliefs. That experience can be related to theories of personal faith development (using the example of Fowler 1981) as well as to more general frameworks of personal development (following a scheme such as that of Erikson 1965).

Bradshaw points out the hidden seductive influence of American theorizing on nursing, a criticism which applies to the social sciences generally, with implications for other aspects of care. The impact of the vast American research and practice establishment upon the rest of the health care world needs to be considered. An analysis by Dueck (1983) suggests that European countries may import ideas from the American world which are not necessarily most relevant to or consistent with European political and social values and institutions, or most pertinent to their epidemiology of illness and philosophy of health care delivery.

To summarize, only recently has 'care' received attention in its own right. Nursing practice and theories of care have been among the most articulated contributions to the care literature, but nursing needs to avoid over-imperialistic claims in this field. The field raises massive issues of personal commitment to care, motivation to undertake the burden of care, ethical values, and the value of persons. Theological concepts of care have an historical endurance which underpin much of our practice unconsciously, and spiritually-framed experiences of care merit closer attention by contemporary care theorists.

References

Blaxter, M. (1976) *The Meaning of Disability: a Sociological Study of Impairment.* Heinemann, London.

Campbell, A.V. (1984) *Moderated love.* SPCK, London.

Cella, D. & Tulsky, D. (1990) Measuring the quality of life today: methodological aspects. *Oncology,* **4**, 29–38.

Downie, R.S. & & Telfer, E. (1980) *Caring and curing.* Methuen, London.

Dueck, A. (1983) American psychology in a cross-cultural context. *Journal of Psychology and Theology,* **11**, 172–80.

Erikson, E. (1965) *Childhood and Society.* Penguin, Harmondsworth.

Finch, J. & Groves, D. (1983) *A Labour of Love: Women, Work, and Caring.* Routledge & Kegan Paul, London.

Fowler, J.W. (1981) *Stages of Faith: the Psychology of Human Developments and the Quest for Meaning.* Harper & Row, San Francisco.

Hall, J.N. (1990) Towards a psychology of caring. *British Journal of Clinical Psychology,* **29**, 129–44.

Halmos, P. (1965) *The Faith of the Counsellors.* Constable, London.

Heasman, K. (1962) *Evangelicalism in Action: an Appraisal of their Social Work in the Victorian Era.* Geoffrey Bles, London.

Hugman, R. (1991) *Power in the Caring Professions.* Macmillan, London.

Kane, R.L. & Kane, R.A. (1982) *Values and Long-term Care.* Lexington Books, Lexington, Massachusetts.

Kitwood, T. (1990) *Concern for Others.* Routledge, London.

McFadyen, A.L. (1990) *The Call to Personhood.* Cambridge University Press, Cambridge.

Nouwen, H.J.M., McNeill, D.P. & Morrison, D.A. (1982) *Compassion.* Darton, Longman and Todd, London.

Oden, T.C. (1983) *Pastoral Theology.* Harper & Row, San Francisco.

Pailin, D.A. (1992) *A gentle touch.* SPCK, London.

Shotter, J. (1980) Men the magicians. In: *Models of Man* (eds A.J. Chapman & D. Jones). British Psychological Society, Leicester.

3 ◆ Patients First: The Obligations of the Subjects of Medical Research

Ruth Chadwick

Medical research poses the problem of potential conflict between the interests of patients (and healthy volunteers) and the interests of society. In this respect it differs from the ethical issues arising in the course of medical therapy. In the latter case there is a presumption that the beneficiary of intervention will be the patient, although others may also be protected (e.g. from infectious disease or from the expression of violence by a person suffering from mental illness), whereas in the case of research it is primarily others who will benefit from the knowledge gained, at least where research is of a nontherapeutic sort. There is thus a potential conflict of interest. 'There should be an intention to benefit society by doing research, and also an obligation to protect subjects of research from harm, and to preserve their rights' (Royal College of Physicians 1986). How is it possible to mediate between these different interests?

This chapter will explore different strategies for dealing with the potential conflict of interest. There is a view that the interests of the subject of research should be given priority, by the protection of the doctrines of informed consent and minimal risk. On the other hand there are arguments for the importance to society of the benefits of medical research. Ways of achieving a balance between the two, by some kind of trade-off between them, will also be examined.

Research and therapy

Although the starting point for the discussion in this chapter was the assumption that there is an essential difference between research and therapy giving rise to ethical issues, it has to be acknowledged that there is by no means a consensus on how the distinction between research and therapy should be drawn. So this is the first issue to be addressed: what is meant by research?

The distinguishing characteristic of research, as opposed to therapy, might be said to lie either in its intention, or in its outcome. The Royal College of Physicians (RCP 1990) takes the first approach, defining research as:

'... where an activity involving a patient is undertaken with the prime purpose of testing a hypothesis and permitting conclusions to be drawn in the hope of contributing to general knowledge'.

Even where therapy is of an innovative kind, it is distinguished from research on the basis of the intention or motive:

> 'In innovative treatment, the sole motive for the action is to choose the best possible course of action for the individual patient even though it be unconventional. It remains innovative treatment rather than research even if, as a byproduct, useful information is gained' (RCP 1990).

The question arises as to whether intention is sufficient as a distinguishing characteristic. Caplan has argued that it is not, that the distinction cannot depend entirely on the health care professional's intentions and that the outcome, or at least the probability of a certain outcome, is also relevant. In particular, it is not possible to classify a procedure as therapy, on the grounds of an intention, if there is little or no evidence to suggest that it will have a therapeutic effect.

Two characteristics that would appear to be especially relevant are the state of knowledge prevailing about the underlying mechanisms or processes that produce a particular result, and the efficacy associated with a particular activity in terms of the probability that it will produce an intended outcome (Caplan 1989).

Yet a third position was taken in the Clothier report on the ethics of gene therapy (Clothier 1992), which classified gene therapy as research rather than innovative treatment. The argument for this position appears to be that gene therapy is *perceived* as different, both in its nature and possible consequences, from treatments used hitherto in medical practice (Clothier 1992). Whether or not it is perceived as different, however, the question remains as to what basis exists for claiming that it really is different. There are good arguments for the view that somatic gene therapy, at least, does not raise issues that are different in principle from conventional forms of medical treatment. Germ-line therapy is more controversial. In the light of uncertainty and of anxieties about possible unforeseen consequences, the Clothier committee's position seems to be connected with the advantages of the possibility for greater regulation that exists when a procedure is classified as research.

The distinction becomes increasingly problematic when the difference between therapeutic and non-therapeutic research is taken into account. Research is classed as therapeutic when 'it is considered that the individual patient might obtain some benefit from participation' (RCP 1990) but where the outcome cannot be guaranteed – otherwise it would not be research. It is interesting to note that the Royal College here uses an outcome-based criterion rather than an intention-based one.

Rather than a sharp dividing line between research and therapy it might be more realistic to think of different points on a continuum:

- non therapeutic research
- therapeutic research

- innovative therapy
- conventional treatment.

It is commonplace that even conventional treatment has an experimental element because every application of a form of treatment is subject to the uniqueness of the individual treated.

At different points on the continuum there will be differences of degree concerning the extent to which there is a probability of benefit to the subject or patient, and the extent to which there is probability of benefits to others as a result of knowledge gained. The important question is how, if at all, it is possible to reconcile the competing interests. This will now be examined from a variety of perspectives: protection of the interests of the subject, the obligation to society, trade-off, weighting strategies, and communitarian ethics.

Protection of the research subject

The history of medical research does not lack examples of horrific abuse of research subjects. Thus it is unsurprising that a popular approach to the potential conflict between the interests of the research subject and those of society is to give priority to the former. This is made explicit in the Clothier report: '... in the sometimes inescapable tensions between the pursuit of knowledge and the protection of patients' interests, the latter must prevail' (Clothier 1992).

The interests of research subjects are normally protected by a combination of the notions of informed consent and of minimal risk. These might be seen as reflections of two of the 'principles of biomedical ethics' (Beauchamp & Childress 1994) – autonomy and non-maleficence, respectively. The question arises, however, as to why informed consent is not sufficient on its own. Why, for example, should informed patients not be free to take even more than minimal risks with their own health, in order to further medical knowledge and thus the good of society? In order to answer this it is necessary to examine both informed consent and minimal risk more closely.

Informed consent

The doctrine of informed consent includes an information-giving component and a voluntariness element. Research subjects must not only be provided with relevant information before agreeing to participate in medical research, but their agreement must also be voluntary, i.e. not as a result of coercion or subtle pressure of some kind. Special safeguards are commonly recommended for vulnerable populations, such as children and persons with a mental disability.

There are reasons for thinking, however, that vulnerability extends beyond these special groups to all research subjects, and that because of the powerful position of the medical researcher vis-à-vis the research subject, the latter always requires extra protection. Eagerness to please the doctor, anxiety that a refusal to participate in a trial might adversely affect one's own treatment, can both have a part to play in enhancing the probability of consent. Hence the desirability of an additional safeguard in the form of a concept of minimal risk.

Even in the case of patients undergoing treatment these arguments have application. The doctor who is acting in the best interests of his or her patient is bound by the principle of nonmaleficence to do no harm, though actions which might count as harm in other, nonmedical contexts might be justified in the course of medical practice in order to produce a therapeutic benefit. So in the doctor–patient relationship, informed consent does not license subjecting the patient to more risk than necessary, because there is an implied promise that the professional is acting in the interests of that patient. There is greater urgency in the research context, however, because as Gillon (1994) has pointed out, that promise is not implied there. The patient bears the risks but others will reap the benefits, if any.

Jonas (1968) goes further, arguing not simply that informed consent needs to be buttressed by the safeguard of minimal risk, but also that even asking people to consent to participate itself undermines the possibility of consent:

> 'The mere issuing of the appeal, the calling for volunteers, with the moral and social pressures it inevitably generates, amounts even under the most meticulous rules of consent to a sort of conscripting'

The problem with this sort of argument is that it seems to follow that nothing would count as consenting to participate in research. He takes the view that it is precisely because of the difficulties inherent in the notion of consent that there is a temptation to turn to other arguments, such as the obligation to society, and yet the dangers in that seem to require the protection of consent:

> 'The awareness of the many ambiguities besetting "consent" actually available and used in medical research prompts recourse to the idea of a public right conceived independently of (and valid prior to) consent; and vice versa, the awareness of the problematic nature of such a right makes even its advocates still insist on the idea of consent with all its ambiguities' (Jonas 1968).

Jonas does have a theory, however, about what would approximate most closely to genuine informed consent, and this is explained in terms of the notion of identification: 'such authentic identification with the cause that it is the subject's as well as the researcher's cause – whereby his role in its service is not just permitted by him, but willed' (Jonas 1968).

It is only this identification that will enable the research subject to avoid becoming an object. Those who can most closely identify are, of course, members of the research community themselves. Outside this there will be a 'descending order' from those who have the greatest access to information and freedom of decision to those who have the least. One of the implications of the principle of identification for patients is that they should only be experimented upon with reference to their own disease.

So both sides of the argument, those supporting individual protection via consent and those supporting the right of society, are problematic. This might lead us to question whether the individual versus society framework is satisfactory. Various responses are possible. The first is to try to bolster the protection of the individual by, for example, the notion of minimal risk. The second is to seek further arguments for the good of the community, as in Jonas' 'sacrificial theme'. Communities have always demanded sacrifices from their members for compelling reasons, e.g. in a state of war. He says: 'We must face the somber truth that the *ultima ratio* of communal life is and always has been the compulsory, vicarious sacrifice of individual lives' (Jonas 1968) and argues that 'something sacrificial' is involved in imposing risks on individuals for a presumed greater common good. A third strategy is to suggest that the opposition between individual and society is misconceived as a conceptual framework to use to address these issues.

Minimal risk

The term minimal risk embraces two situations:

> '... where the level of psychological or physical distress is negligible though there may be a small chance of a reaction which is itself trivial, e.g. a mild headache or feeling of lethargy. The second is where there is a very remote chance of serious injury or death, comparable to the risk of flying as a passenger on a scheduled aircraft' (RCP 1990).

In other words, it can apply to the content of a risk or to the probability of a risk, where in the latter case the content can be very great.

There are clearly questions about what, in numerical terms, counts as a 'very remote' risk, and some might want to argue that it is never acceptable to expose a research subject to a risk of death, however remote. There is a further problem, however, about how people interpret risk, and whether what seems remote to one person also appears remote to another. If those problems can be solved, much may depend on how the information is presented. Adopting a policy of minimal risk rather than, for example, one of maximizing expected utility, is a way of prioritizing the interests of the patient over society. But should they be given absolute priority? Is there to be no trade-off between the policy of minimal risk and the interests of society?

Obligations to society

As stated above, Jonas acknowledges that there may be reasons of a compelling sort for communities or societies to demand sacrifices from their members. He denies, however, that the benefits to be gained from medical research are of a compelling sort. Against this Ackerman (1993) has argued that there are categories of obligation regarding the general welfare similar to those of individual beneficence, and that these generate duties in the context of medical research. The use of the term 'duties' is significant: he is making a stronger claim than that it is desirable to conduct research to expand knowledge.

Ackerman takes the view that Jonas' argument relies on questionable assumptions, e.g. that there is a moral difference between causing harm and failing to prevent it, so that it is not as bad to fail to do medical research which will lead to the minimization of suffering as it is to cause harm by active means. People can be helped by doing medical research, and if we fail to facilitate such help we are harming them. But who exactly are the beneficiaries of the duties argued for by Ackerman? Those who will benefit most directly are future patients, who may even be future, i.e. as yet unborn, people. In the case of the latter there are particular philosophical problems as to whether it is possible to argue that there are obligations to people who do not yet exist. Even if there are, it is not clear how they should be weighed against obligations to currently existing people.

Medical research will not benefit future people only, however. The beneficiaries of medical research may be existing people who will become patients in 20 years' time. Further, there are the more intangible benefits that accrue to all who live in a society in which forward-looking research is being done.

If we accept that there are obligations to carry out medical research, but that there must also be some limits to the sacrifices that can be expected (or even allowed) of individuals, then there has to be some strategy for achieving a balance between the different considerations.

Trade-off

In a trade-off situation the benefits of doing research are traded against the risks imposed on the subjects. A simple form of trade-off would be a numerical one: if a sufficient number of people could be helped by doing the research, it would be justified to expose a small number of individuals to risk. Support for such a strategy would depend on the assumption that the interests on either side of the equation carried equal weight. This kind of numerical trade-off on its own has clear dangers: it only too readily lends credence to Jonas' idea that individuals are in danger of being 'sacrificed' for the good of the majority.

An alternative suggestion concerns the situation where the *degree* of potential benefit is sufficiently large, although this might be combined with a point about the number of people who could be helped or harmed. The Royal College of Physicians acknowledges that there may be situations where the expected benefits are so great that a larger than minimal risk is acceptable. The more obvious situation is where the great potential benefit is to the person who is actually undergoing risk, but there may be rare situations in which nontherapeutic research involving greater than minimal risk is justified (RCP 1990). While their view seems to allow the possibility for trade-off, depending on the assessment of the degree of benefit to be gained, they do not, however, make clear what would count as an example of such a situation.

From time to time there is reported in the media an account of a patient who has reached a last though very slim chance of life. In such a situation it is sometimes argued that to carry out a very experimental therapy is justifiable – it is their only chance, and while the intervention in question is very unlikely to help them it may produce knowledge which will help others in future. This argument was used both in the Laura Davies case, where a young girl was subject to multiple organ transplants, and in the Cline affair, when Martin Cline tried gene therapy without approval, subsequently losing his research funding. In both cases the use of the argument was the subject of considerable controversy.

A risk greater than minimal is said by the Royal College of Physicians not to be acceptable where the research subjects are healthy volunteers (RCP 1986). Why is this? Presumably because, while it may be unlikely that patients will benefit, it is not even considered to be a possibility that healthy volunteers will benefit by participating in medical research. This makes it clear that the position of the Royal College is not really a trade-off position after all; they are not willing to trade more than minimal risks to subjects against potential benefits unless there is also a possibility of benefit for the subjects themselves. This issue is linked with that of the status of the volunteer and the availability of compensation, which will be considered below.

The presumptive weighting strategy

An alternative to the simple trade-off view is the sort of weighting strategy suggested by Ackerman (1993). As he points out, the policy of giving absolute priority to the interests of research subjects is itself a weighting strategy, as is the use of the doctrines of informed consent and minimal risk to protect research subjects. The kind of weighting he favours, however, which he calls 'the presumptive weighting strategy', is one that recognizes competing duties, but not in equal proportion. Presumptive priority is assigned to duties to subjects, requiring their full satisfaction in most circumstances. However, this presumption may be overridden if it is necessary to undertake research activities that may prevent or remove important harms to others and there will be no more than minor compromises in protections for the interests of subjects.

According to Ackerman this strategy has several advantages: recognition of the pre-eminence of the interests of subjects; acknowledgement of the 'duties of rescue in the research context', i.e., the importance of carrying out research to prevent avoidable harm, and an accompanying recognition of the justifiability of imposing some risks on subjects; and restricting compromises of research subjects to the minimum necessary.

It might appear that in practice this presumptive weighting strategy would amount to the protection of research subjects by the doctrines of informed consent and minimal risk with which we started. But the strategy as Ackerman has described it allows room for interpretation and demands judgement. Thus it is not simply an application of certain doctrines.

> 'Key phrases, such as "minor compromises in the requirements of duties to subjects" ... require interpretation. Concern may arise about excessive latitude in determining compromises in the interests of subjects. However, a more rigid approach prevents proper recognition of duties of rescue in the research setting. Thus this latitude is inescapable if our weighting strategy is to acknowledge fully all dimensions of the moral landscape' (Ackerman, 1993)

There is a contrast with the approach of the Royal College described above, which also calls for the exercise of judgment but which, as we have seen, takes a very rigid approach to research on healthy volunteers.

Compensation strategies and communitarianism

Another way of mediating between the interests of the research subject and the interests of society is by offering compensation for harm, notably of a 'no-fault' kind. There have been calls for no-fault compensation for the victims of harm in the course of medical research, although why such people should be treated differently from patients harmed in the course of medical treatment is not always clear (Harvey & Chadwick 1992).

Compensation could be viewed either as a strengthening or a watering down of patient protection. If interpreted as an addition to the requirements of informed consent and minimal risk, it would be a strengthening – patients should be protected by provision of clear information, absence of pressure, the assurance that risks will be minimal, and, if anything should go wrong, by compensation without recourse to the law of tort. On the other hand, the availability of compensation might be seen as a threat to the protection of minimal risk, by increasing the likelihood that researchers will be willing to engage in research that does involve greater than minimal risk.

One of the principal arguments given for availability of no-fault compensation is in terms of fairness. The Royal College of Physicians report *Research Involving Patients* says 'there is an element of benefit to society and it seems fair that society should bear some of the risk in financial terms' (RCP 1990).

As Harvey and Chadwick have pointed out, however:

> 'This idea that some individuals' gains are at the expense of others'

losses (which need to be made good) serve to emphasize the element of conflict between the interests of different individuals. Such an emphasis is common in an atomistic view of society. There is another view which sees the interest of individuals as being much more closely interconnected (Harvey & Chadwick 1992).

This point might be developed in different ways. First, it might be argued that there are indirect benefits for all individuals in living in a society in which research is being conducted. *Research Involving Patients* points to 'the benefit of the addition to general knowledge which would be to the advantage of all patients in the long run' (RCP 1990). Second, it could be said that to interpret the issue as a conflict between the competing interests of different individuals is the wrong way to look at it. From a communitarian perspective the very identity of the individual is partly constituted as a member of a community. For communitarians, the fundamental values are the communal ones such as solidarity. They will support actions that promote the common good and traditional practices and which involve the exercise of co-operative virtues (Beauchamp & Childress 1994).

How might this perspective be applied in the current context? Members of the community, in expressing solidarity with one another, will help those in need, which might involve making compensation available to those who have been harmed (but this would be applicable not only to the victims of research but also to patients harmed in the course of medical treatment); they will also, however, arguably have positive obligations to promote the common good by providing the opportunity to develop techniques for helping victims of disease, and this will require research to be carried out. From this perspective, the theme of 'demanding' sacrifice from individuals should be replaced by one of a sense of responsibility for the common good. This, moreover, is in accordance with Jonas' requirements for his principle of identification, which appeals to 'the one, mysterious, and sacred source of ... generosity of the will – "devotion", whose forms and objects of commitment are various' (Jonas 1968).

Conclusions

The variety of strategies examined for mediating between the interests of research subjects and of the community have differed largely in the degree to which they give weight to one over the other. Consideration of compensation policies and of communitarianism, however, suggests that it may be unwise to begin from the point of view that these different interests are necessarily in competition.

Another point to emerge from the discussion is the difficulty of laying down hard and fast rules. Different areas may demand exercise of judgement in different ways. As mentioned above, for example, the Clothier committee, in the report on the ethics of gene therapy, recommended that this therapy be treated as research. Despite this they say that the purpose of somatic gene therapy is 'to alleviate disease in that individual, and that individual alone' (Clothier 1992). Germ-line gene therapy is ruled out at present on the grounds that there is insufficient knowledge to evaluate the risks to future generations. Thus, although as we have seen throughout the discussion above, the central ethical issue in research is how to balance the interests of research subjects against the interests of potential (other) beneficiaries, the Clothier committee classifies gene therapy as research while wanting to restrict its use to attempts to benefit the individual alone. It remains true, however, that knowledge will be gained in the course of such therapy which will benefit other people and the possibility is left open that at some future date germ-line therapy may also be acceptable.

So where does the above discussion leave the subject of research? It is fashionable nowadays to stress responsibilities as well as rights, even outside the ranks of those who would class themselves as communitarians. From that point of view individual patients, as well as society as a whole, would have a responsibility to promote the common good. Does this imply that there is an *obligation* to participate? Rather, it is a shift in the *presumption* regarding the balance of interests. The freedom to refuse would be set against a background of a sense of social responsibility, rather than in the context of rights above all. In this case the need for additional safeguards such as minimal risk would be clearer than when set alongside the informed consent requirement in the context of a more individualistic view.

Reading guide

Jonas, H. (1968) Philosophical reflections on human experimentation. *Daedalus*, 219–45. RCP (1986) *Research on Healthy Volunteers*. Royal College of Physicians, London.

RCP (1990) *Research Involving Patients*. Royal College of Physicians, London.

References

Ackerman, T. (1993) Medical research, society and health care ethics. In: *Principles of Health Care Ethics* (ed. R. Gillon). Wiley, Chichester.

Beauchamp, T.G. & Childress, J.F. (1994) *Principles of Biomedical Ethics*, 4th edn. Oxford University Press, New York.

Caplan, A. (1989) Arguing with success: is in vitro fertilization research or therapy? In: *Beyond Baby M* (eds D. Bartels *et al.*) Humana Press, Clifton, New Jersey.

Clothier, C.M. (Chairman) (1992) *Report of the Committee on the Ethics of Gene Therapy*. HMSO, London.

Gillon, R. (1994) Paper presented at the Second World Congress of the International Association of Bioethics, Buenos Aires.

Harvey, I. & Chadwick, R. (1992) Compensation for harm: the implications for medical research. *Social Science and Medicine*, **34** (12), 1399–404.

Jonas, H. (1968) Philosophical reflections on human experimentation. *Daedalus*, 219–45.

Commentary on Chapter 3

Margaret Brazier

The title of Chadwick's analysis of the conflicts of interest inherent in clinical research rings alarm bells in the mind of the lawyer. *Obligations of subjects of medical research* suggests that participation in research may somehow be mandatory! The citizen is obliged to pay her taxes. Is she to be obliged to lend her body to promote the common good? However, Chadwick's meticulous analysis of the competing interests in the regulation of research reveals a picture fundamentally reflecting for the most part the current state of English law.

The interests of research subjects, Chadwick asserts, are normally protected by notions of informed consent and minimal risk. Those ethical imperatives are mirrored by the law. Research on a competent patient will be unlawful unless he is fully informed (1) of the fact that doctors seek to enrol him in a research trial, and (2) of all the material hazards inherent in participation in the trial. In the context of clinical research it probably does not matter that in *Sidaway* v. *Royal Bethlem Hospital* (1985) the House of Lords adopted the professional, rather than the patient standard, to judge the adequacy of information offered to patients receiving treatment. The profession in the promulgation of its own guidelines on research (RCP 1989) and the Department of Health (DoH 1991) have made it crystal clear that, whatever the case in relation to treatment, fully informed consent is required from research subjects (Brazier 1992).

Minimal risk is a little more problematic for the lawyer. The researcher desiring to carry out research using any vertebrate animal must be licensed to do so under the Animals (Scientific Procedures) Act 1986. He must satisfy a Home Office inspector that the risk and pain to the animal are justified by the potential benefit ensuing from his research. No analogous legislation controls research on human subjects. However, within the NHS any research proposal must be approved by a local research ethics committee. A researcher seeking to evade such vetting of his proposal could be disciplined by her employer. Outside the NHS, the Royal College of Physicians has made it clear that a failure to seek ethical scrutiny of a research programme could constitute professional misconduct. Regulating research by means of a nonstatutory review system is far from ideal, but the law and practice recognise society's obligations to attempt to protect research subjects.

Chadwick's chapter goes further than this, considering the impact of concepts of communitarianism in relation to research. Does the law acknowledge any such concept? The answer is yes, but to a limited extent. In 1978 the Royal Commission on Civil Liability (Pearson 1978) recommended that Parliament should legislate to ensure that any research subject who suffered injury as a result of participation in a clinical trial received compensation for her injury on a no-fault basis. The Commission argued that a citizen who endangers her own health for the good of the community was entitled to the support of the community if she suffered harm. Parliament has never legislated to that effect, but increasingly in drug trials at least the principle is endorsed by the creation by the pharmaceutical company of a no-fault compensation scheme. Many local research ethics committees insist that such provision is made for compensation before approving a research protocol.

The community's obligations to the subjects are recognized, if imperfectly, by the law. Are obligations *to* the community on the part of the subject given any legal credence? The recent proposals for reform of the law relating to mentally incapacitated patients (Law Commission 1995) appear to do so. No competent patient may be conscripted into a research programme. Chadwick and I are free to reject any plea that we exercise altruism for the benefit of society. Where a person is incapable, by reason of mental disability, of giving her own consent to participate in clinical research, the legality of any such research has been dubious in the extreme. Treatment of an adult patient incapable of giving an independent consent has been held to be lawful if found to be in his best interests and in conformity to good medical practice (*F* v. *West Berkshire HA* 1989). When an incompetent patient was enrolled in a therapeutic research trial, it was argued that the prospect of benefit was sufficient to render the procedure in his interests and so lawful. In a nontherapeutic trial no such argument could hold water. Yet knowledge of certain diseases, such as Alzheimer's, probably could not be expanded without some form of research on current sufferers for the benefit of future generations.

The Law Commission has given its support for a formal measure of law reform which largely reflects the present practice of many ethics committees. They recommend that:

'... research which is unlikely to benefit a participant, or whose benefit is likely to be long delayed, should be lawful in relation to a person without capacity to consent if (1) the research is into an incapacitating condition with which the participant is or may be affected and (2) certain statutory procedures are complied with'.

The statutory procedures include the following. A national mental incapacity research committee would review all protocols involving incompetent subjects. That committee must satisfy itself of the benefit of the proposed research, that the object of the research cannot be achieved without the participation of incompetent subjects, and that the research will not involve 'more than negligible risk, will not be unduly invasive or restrictive of a participant and will not unduly interfere with a participant's freedom of action or privacy'. In addition to the approval of the mental incapacity research committee, no individual can be enrolled in a trial without either court approval, or the consent of his nominated proxy or manager (in effect his guardian), or a certificate from a doctor not involved in the research that the individual's participation is appropriate, or designation that the research does not involve direct contact.

The Law Commission has expressly sought to effect a compromise between the interests of research subjects and the interests of the community. Measures are taken to attempt to safeguard the subject from any significant harm or distress. Yet the basic premise is that there is some degree of obligation to the community. Interestingly that obligation is not to the community as a whole. Only research of possible benefit to those who share the subject's affliction will be allowed. Rightly, patients unable to consent on their own behalf and so protect their own interests, are not made the means of achieving society's wider health care ends. But should the Law Commission have gone as far as it has done? I may take the benefit of research on others without any reciprocal obligation on my part. A patient with Alzheimer's or an adult with Down's syndrome will, if the Law Commission's proposals become law, in effect be conscripted for the common good.

References

Brazier, M. (1992) *Medicine, Patients and the Law*, 2nd edn, Chapter 19. Penguin, Harmondsworth.

DoH (1991) Local Research Ethics Committees. HMSO, London.

F v. *West Berkshire Health Authority* (1989) 2 *All England Reports* 545, HL.

Law Commission (1995) Report No 231, *Mental Incapacity*. HMSO, London.

Pearson (1978) *Royal Commission on Civil Liability and Compensation for Personal Injury*. Cmnd 7054, paras 1340–41. HMSO, London.

RCP (1989) *Guidelines on the Practice of Ethics Committees in Research Involving Human Subjects*, 2nd ed. Royal College of Physicians, London.

Sidaway v. *Royal Bethlem Hospital* (1985) 1 *All England Reports* 643, HL.

4 ◆ Ethnography and the Development of Patient-Centred Nursing

Steven Ersser

Improvements in our ability to develop patient-centred health care are to some extent dependent on our capacity to understand and respond to the patient's experience of care. Ethnographic research offers a systematic and rigorous way of examining this experience, through offering description and explanation of the 'insider's' viewpoint. Ethnographic accounts can highlight the subtle features of those familiar aspects of social life often taken for granted. These may help us to re-examine health care by revealing the unexpected. In this chapter I will highlight the value of using an interpretative research approach to raise awareness of patient-centred nursing, using ethnographic data from a study of the therapeutic effect of nursing. This study is described in more detail in Ersser (1991, 1995).

Outline of an ethnographic study of nursing

Ethnography is an approach to qualitative research which is used to describe and analyse the way of life of a particular culture or cultural groups (Germain 1986). This interpretive approach is concerned with understanding social life from the perspective of those being studied (Spradley 1979). An assumption underlying ethnographic research is that people's actions are influenced by the interpretation or sense they make of situations.

The aim of the study was to identify and describe the views of both hospital nurses and adult patients with regard to the beneficial and adverse effects of nursing. The study involved 17 cases, ten nurses and seven patients. Fieldwork was conducted in four wards in three hospitals within the same health authority. One ward specialised in neurology, one in dermatology, and the remainder were general medical wards.

Three methods of data collection were used:

(1) Semi-structured self-administered diaries which were completed by both nurses and patients in the study.
(2) 'Ethnographic' interviews (semi-structured in-depth interviews used to determine cultural knowledge) involving patients and nurses.
(3) Group discussions (for nurse participants only).

Data collection was initiated using the following question, either through use of a group discussion and then a diary (nurses) or the diary (patients):

'I am interested in your experience of giving (nurses)/receiving (patients) nursing care. In particular I would like you to try and describe how you believe the nursing you give (nurses)/receive (patients) affects your patient/you.'

This statement was written on a diary instruction sheet. Participants were given up to five days to keep the diary. The interviews were used to allow the participants to elaborate and clarify issues raised in the group discussion or diary. The types of question asked included those which allowed the participant to describe the context of their situation, and questions to determine and distinguish the various categories of interpretation of the nurse's action and its consequences.

The study also involved the use of a grounded theory approach, which is a method of data collection and analysis used to develop social theory (Glaser 1978). Data analysis include the use of a process of content analysis and a comparison across all the sets of data to reveal the various categories of data.

In the course of this research a great quantity of data was collected on patients' experiences and views of the nursing they received, and on nurses' reflections on their interactions with patients. The excerpts of data used are mainly derived from the diaries and interviews.

In this chapter I will emphasize those aspects of nursing which patients considered to be important, whether or not nurses saw these aspects as important. A truly patient-centred approach to nursing must take very seriously the patient experience of nursing care. The nursing perspective will also be illustrated. Data excerpts from the interviews with patients and nurses have been selected as being typical and faithful to the emphasis given in the accounts. The participants' names have been changed in order to preserve anonymity.

Overview of patients' and nurses' views

There were a number of aspects of nursing care which both patients and nurses viewed as important. Significant emphasis was given to the expressive or personal aspects of nursing; that is, reference to *how* the nurse acts (the presentation of the nurse). This includes:

● the nurse's personal qualities, including attitude, manner, personality, facial expression and appearance (the nurse as a person);

- the importance of the nurse being with the patient and readily available for the patient (the presence of the nurse).

However, the importance given by nurses and patients to some features of nursing differed; for example, patients emphasized the effect of nurses' moods, of their feeling tired, of their instilling confidence and providing humour, to a much greater extent than did nurses. Patients also highlighted the importance of the nurse's facial expression. Nurses emphasized the importance of introducing themselves to patients to a greater extent than did patients. Further illustrations are given later (excerpts 12 and 13).

Some specific examples of patients' and nurses' views

I will focus on a number of specific issues identified as important by patients, illustrated using some data on the presentation of the nurse. A patient-centred approach to nursing requires recognition of the importance of these specific issues to patients. I will organize these specific illustrations under a number of general subheadings.

(1) *Conveying to the patient that they are valued*

A patient on the dermatology ward emphasizes the importance of the nurse accepting them with their disfigurement.

Excerpt 1 – Patient

'They're so used to skin things – they don't say "disgusting" or something just because you've got it. The main problem is being out and about, because the skin problem is the sort of thing that people wouldn't think you would have to go into hospital for, because it doesn't kill you or anything. People don't realise how important it is to have clear skin and it does make a difference, not just socially but mentally. You know because you can't go swimming say or you feel uncomfortable with your friends. I mean the summer is worse obviously because you can't wear the clothes you would like to wear. But it's not just that it's uncomfortable – a lot of people get it (psoriasis) so that it cracks and that sort of thing...'

The next excerpt reinforces the failure of nurses to treat the patient as 'a person'. This patient suffered from motor neurone disease and had a new tracheostomy.

Excerpt 2 - Patient

Patient: 'Two nurses came in. I think it was to take my clothes off to be examined by the doctor. They just came in and totally ignored me, they treated me like I wasn't really there, just kind of took off my clothes and talked over me. I mean, in situations where nurses are doing personal things and actually chatting away ... I think it's usually when they don't know you and perhaps they are used to dealing with a lot of disabled people, who maybe can't communicate. I suppose that when I start to talk and show that I am a person and not someone who can't communicate, then they have to respond to me.

Interviewer: 'When these two nurses were talking over you what was going through your mind?'

Patient: 'Horror! You know just feeling horror and angry as well... You always feel like you can't afford to get mad at them because you're dependent on them.'

The nurse's facial expression is also seen to have meaning and consequences for the patient. The next account is given by an elderly woman who had a prolonged hospital stay, few visitors and limited mobility.

Excerpt 3 – Patient

Interviewer: 'You referred, Nina, to the nurse Sally. You said "neither a smile, nor a word, nor even a look"' (interrupted).

Patient: 'Oh yes, I remember she used to come and do things and neither look at me, nor smile, nor speak. And that's not nice for a patient you know. It makes you feel as if you're of no consequence, you know what I mean?'

(2) The importance of the nurse's presence: being there and being available

The data highlights the importance patients and nurses place on the nurse being with the patient at certain key times, physically and psychologically. It is easy for a nurse to think that they are not doing anything when, for example, simply accompanying a patient who is due to have an investigation to the X-ray department. However this study strongly suggests that the presence of a nurse can be of great importance to the patient.

Features of the nurse's presence described by patients and nurses include the nurse's sensitivity to the patient's viewpoint, and the nurse being caring and conveying to the patient that they have time for them. Only nurses made direct reference to the importance of 'being with' the patient and providing 'support'.

Excerpt 4 – Patient

Patient: 'They have time for you and I think all patients just want to have time.'

Interviewer: 'Does that affect you in some way when you feel nurses are giving you time?'

Patient: 'Yes, you don't feel nervous about asking them. If, you say "would you do so and so for me now", they say "don't hesitate to ask". Now if it was somebody who was short tempered or you weren't keen on – I mean you can't like everyone the same can you – you'd hesitate about asking them. I wouldn't separate anybody here, I would ask any of them.... They never seem to rush you.'

The following illustrates how the nurse's presence is believed to help a patient cope with an investigation.

Excerpt 5 – Nurse

'Today I went down for an investigation with a lady and she had to wait around and so I went back to the ward. I said I'd try and get back there, and she was really keen that I should. When I came in she was having an endoscopy and she was really anxious and wasn't breathing well; they'd already started when I got there. And as soon as I was there she sort of calmed down a lot and then she said afterwards, "I was so glad you came in, I knew you were going to come, you wouldn't let me down" ... I mean I wasn't doing anything, just being with this patient.'

The inability of nurses to convey their presence with the patient may be seen to have an adverse effect. Here a patient with a new tracheostomy became anxious with the long absence of the nurse, for fear of having another respiratory arrest.

Excerpt 6 –Patient

'I mean sometimes I'm just sort of on the loo and my chest's a bit rough, I know somebody might not come for a while, you know, it takes a lot of confidence to sit there, particularly bearing in mind I did have a ... I did stop breathing and I did have a bout in ITU and it was bound to have some effect on me. You know, I need to build up my confidence – you know that does take ... ermm, quite an effort on my part, just to, you know relax and realise that nothing is going to happen.'

The difficulty experienced by nurses in giving patients sufficient time was given some emphasis in their accounts.

Excerpt 7 – Nurse

'I spoke about Verena yesterday. When I came on duty she was still looking very ill, and the doctors had discontinued all treatment. Her son was actually with her, which was good for her ... Verena's son disappeared off the ward shortly after I came on duty. Verena was quite distressed and kept calling for me by name. At the time all I wanted to do was go and sit with her and talk to her, but just couldn't as we had all the drugs to hand out and everyone to settle – what do you do? Eventually we asked an auxiliary from the next ward to come and sit with Verena until her son returned. Verena continued to call for me and then asked for the injection she had the night before (diamorph.) to help her sleep. She finally went to sleep sitting in her chair and never woke up. I felt bad because all the time I was talking to her son – and she was all on her own when she died ... I felt Verena really would have appreciated me being there and I had let her down.'

The nurse's presence is seen by some patients to provide reassurance and comfort.

Excerpt 8 – Patient

'I am writing from my bed ... First, I attend this hospital every four weeks for blood, and the care and attention I receive is the best from all doctors and nurses. Comfort is a number one presently. I get it all the time. Also a nurse

will sit and talk to you if you have any worries – which I find a great help.
Also, ring the bell and help is quickly at hand. ...'

Through showing an effort to give the patient time the nurse was seen
to help create a more relaxed environment, and the patient to feel
valued as a person.

Excerpt 9 – Patient
This patient contrasts her experience on a surgical ward with that on a
dermatology ward. She is beginning to talk of her expectations of
nurses.

> *Patient:* 'Well, on other wards I've been on, like surgical wards, they usually
> come in and they chat but they usually have to rush off a lot more ... In all
> professions time is always the thing that is expensive. In a surgical ward
> there are dressings to change – they don't have the time they are allowed
> here. Even if they are busy, they can manage to give you more time I think.'
> *Interviewer:* 'I was going to ask you what effect that has on you?'
> *Patient:* 'I think it is relaxing because you don't feel that they are so rushed,
> even if they're busy, because they are giving time – rather than "Oh I've got
> to do this, got to do that." That's more relaxing for you.'

(Expanding on this later)

> 'It's nice that people sit and do that (give you time) you feel like you're sort of
> a person, rather than just a patient or a number or a name – the fact that they
> take time to sit down and talk to you and answer things.'

Excerpt 10 – Nurse

> *Nurse:* 'We can listen to their fears whereas the doctors can't stand there for a
> long time. It might take a long time for something to come out of a patient
> and often when you're doing the dressing or treatment they're talking to you
> and little things come out ... It helps them relax more because if you rush
> them they won't tell you anything because they can see you're in a hurry to
> get out ...'
> *Interviewer:* 'How do you do that?'
> *Nurse:* 'It's hard, it's something that comes I think. Sitting down when all the
> time I'd like to be standing up – edging to the door, because I know there's
> something else out there I should be going.'

Despite the difficulty of being available for patients, nurses show a
variety of ways in which they attempt to convey their presence to
patients, for example:

Excerpt 11 – Nurse

> 'It's making people feel at ease on the one level, but on another level if you
> can – as when I said to people not to be afraid to ask – I'm showing them that
> I am actually available, that they shouldn't. ... I mean you will actually get
> patients who'll come in and they'll sit there all day and they're uncomfor-
> table and they won't say. If I'm actually telling them that I'm available and I
> don't mind, then they're much more willing to actually ask for the help they
> need.'

(3) *Involving the patient in their health care: the importance of discrepancies between nurse and patient views*

An important feature of ethnographic data is that it provides an opportunity to compare professional and lay perspectives (Ragucci 1972). This is illustrated in those accounts where nurses emphasize the importance of giving patients choice, whereas patients are perhaps more ambivalent. This example is an important one because many nurses view patient involvement in their care as a patient-centred practice. The following excerpts illustrate the problem.

Excerpt 12 – Nurse
(Discussing the ward's 'nursing approach')

'It's very geared towards the education of nurses and the involvement of patients ... I think they feel more involved in the actual care and they don't feel just another patient that's a number or a bed or a condition ... For one thing it makes them feel more comfortable in the ward situation. It makes them feel more willing to ask questions.'

Excerpt 13 – Nurse

Nurse: 'I tried to encourage independence by asking Chris to get his things together to wash. He appeared to be unhappy about this and said he felt I was being bossy.'

(Expanding on this later)

Nurse: 'I think he thought "Oh sod her, I'm not doing it anyway".'
Interviewer: 'If a patient does perceive you as bossy, what effect do you think that has on them? Does it have any effect on them.'
Nurse: 'Well, patients are all individuals and some people like being bossed, some people think "oh well, great somebody is making me do something at last, I'm not just sitting here doing nothing" ... They don't like this wishy washy "What do you feel you might be able to do, Mr so and so?" Other patients absolutely hate it.'

The literature on patient-centred care does not adequately account for patients' perceptions (as illustrated in Brearley 1990). The findings from this study are consistent with those of Waterworth and Luker (1990), and indicate that some patients may in fact be 'reluctant collaborators'.

Ethnographic data: a pointer to patient-centred health care

Patient-centred nursing depends upon nurses having a sufficient awareness of patients' cultural differences. Ethnography can raise appreciation of different cultural perspectives (Dobson 1986; Burrows 1983) including the subtle variations found among people from the same broad cultural grouping, e.g. Cornwell's (1984) study. The ethnographic approach specifically allows cultural knowledge to be identified; this is useful because much of the knowledge which informs our social actions is taken for granted. This may include, for example, the value of being with another person during times of distress.

Ethnographic research has validity advantages compared to approaches such as surveys, because of the commitment and means to understand the viewpoint of others. This includes, for example, the closeness of the researcher to the social situation under study, which enables data to be generated which is meaningful to patients and health care staff. Also, careful attention is paid to understanding the context in which patient accounts are given, and presenting this context to enhance data validity. This is illustrated by Excerpt 6 above, highlighting the importance of the nurse's presence to a patient who had previously suffered a respiratory arrest.

Ethnography is particularly useful when exploratory work is necessary; for example, it may be premature to conduct a patient satisfaction survey without having obtained sufficient information upon which to construct valid questions. There is a danger of conducting a questionnaire survey framed in terms of what health care staff assume to be relevant to patients.

Interpretive research provides a basis for making transparent the subtle meanings found in communication (Fay 1975). The way in which the nurse's actions convey to the patient that they are valued is illustrated in Excerpts 1–3. This data offers an opportunity to change the way we view familiar situations. Even when health care staff have a sense of the importance of subtle changes in the language and actions of patients, these can be difficult to discuss effectively. Ethnographic interviews provide a basis for patients and health staff to explore and communicate their experience. Also, the grounded theory approach permits the identification and labelling of taken-for-granted or hidden concepts in health care situations. This is exemplified by the concept of the nurse's presence.

The educational value of ethnographic data is apparent from the illustrations given. It also has a use in health policy research (Strong & Robinson 1988). However, care is needed in the use of such findings, which are appropriately seen only as pointers for reflection, rather than prescriptions for action.

The value of the process of ethnographic research

The experience of engaging in ethnographic research can provide opportunities for developing patient-centred health care. The nurses in this study found that keeping a diary and being interviewed helped them to develop their awareness of their conduct and its implications for patients.

Excerpt 14 – Nurse

'The idea of individualized patient care really appealed to me. It's taken a long time but I suppose I still like being in charge; but I'd rather look after my patients – because of that I'm not bored with nursing any more ... I just felt very bad about the way I was nursing my patients because I wasn't caring for them as I should have been. It was just a job. It was only because of circumstance. Just before you'd asked that question I'd had some time off and I'd been thinking about it and suddenly realised why I was feeling like this and so I'd just started to change my attitude.'

After interview this nurse recounted how the study helped her to address the conflict she experienced between her beliefs about patient-centred care and the reality of her practice as a staff nurse.

The personal and social aspects of research activity are important to the outcome of the research (Newby 1977; Bell & Roberts 1984). As a nurse and researcher my own involvement in ethnographic research helped to deepen my knowledge of patient-centred nursing for use on return to clinical practice and teaching.

Some sociologists regard social research methods as refinements of the methods we employ in everyday life to understand the world (Hammersley & Atkinson 1983). The ethnographic approach raises important questions about how valid information is obtained from patients in health care situations using different methods.

Patient reactions to involvement in ethnographic research

The open-ended diary question allowed patients a high degree of freedom to refer to issues of personal relevance at a time and in a way which suited their preference. This is often not possible with use of a questionnaire. Despite initial uncertainty by patients about their ability to write something useful in their diary, most managed to use it for the suggested five days. Arrangements were discussed with the patient and senior nurse on the ward about withdrawing should they feel too tired, unwell or burdened. Invariably the diary provided a useful basis for clarifying and exploring patient experiences through the subsequent interviews.

The use of diaries and interviewing as evaluative tools within health care is underdeveloped. Such methods have advantages over methods such as questionnaires, because they often give participants greater opportunity and flexibility to communicate. Also, the methodical but informal style of the ethnographic interview helped to develop the trust necessary to allow patients to express views, including their criticisms.

Consideration needs to be given to the potential for intrusion which some may experience through the use of interpretive research methods. It has been argued that systematic attempts to examine the viewpoints of others within modern organizations ('subjectification') is a way of extending medical power (Foucault 1986). A parallel may be drawn with nurses' initiatives to develop patient-centred nursing through making greater efforts to get to know and relate to patients (Armstrong 1983; May 1992) and their involvement in observation and bodily care (Lawler 1991). However, counter-arguments suggest that such 'surveillance' can be enabling (Giddens in Bryant & Jary 1991). In practice I found patients invariably valued and enjoyed the opportunity to talk during the interviews. Comparable observations have been made by other ethnographers (Wax 1971).

The limitations of ethnographic data

The effort invested in the collection and analysis of ethnographic data warrants some attention to its limitations. Contention surrounds the degree to which ethnographic accounts legitimately claim to represent an independent social reality, and the extent to which they enable us to capture something of this reality more accurately than other approaches. Hammersley (1992) challenges the realist conception of validity, arguing that rather than representing reality, ethnographic accounts simply construct versions of reality. He suggests that we recognize that accounts are selective constructions without rejecting the idea that they may represent phenomena independent of themselves and of the researcher, more or less accurately. Doyal (1993) calls for caution on the adoption of relativist approaches to the development of knowledge relevant to nursing, especially in the area of ethics where he argues that consideration of universal needs and cultural neutrality are important.

Conclusions

Both the process and product of ethnographic research may be helpful in understanding health care from the patient's perspective. In this chapter I have used data collected in the course of an ethnographic study to illustrate some aspects of nursing care which are seen by patients and nurses as important. Ethnography offers a basis to challenge beliefs and practices which are organized for the convenience of professionals or the organization. A wide range of data collection methods should be used to obtain valid evaluative information on patient experience. However, qualitative research approaches must not be seen as a simple and quick alternative to quantitative methods. Indeed, efforts to record the patient's experience of health care in a highly valid way require both the analysis and presentation of such data to be rigorous. Ethnographic data may also be helpful for the purposes of education and policy review. Ethnographic research could contribute to the development of a professional discourse which is based on a fuller recognition of the patient's interpretation of health care.

Reading guide

Helpful introductions to the use of ethnography as a research approach are provided by Fetterman (1989) and Atkinson (1979). A practical guide to conducting ethnographic interviews is provided by Spradley (1979). More detail on theoretical issues can be found in the chapters by

Aamodt, Lipson and Field in Morse (1991). The debate on the contribution of social constructionism to development of medical sociology is provided by Bury (1986). His work is illustrated in Bury (1988). Hammersley (1992) offers a useful critical guide to reading ethnographic research. Readable illustrations of ethnographic studies in health care include Germain (1979) and Cornwell (1984). A critical review of much of the literature relating to patient-centred nursing, with a specific focus on the organization of nursing work, is provided by Ersser and Tutton (1991). Fitzpatrick and Hopkins (1983) have written a helpful paper on the conceptual issues related to patient satisfaction research. Health related ethnographic studies and methodological issues may be found in the journal *Qualitative Health Research* (Sage Publications).

References

Armstrong, D. (1983) The fabrication of nurse–patient relationships. *Social Science and Medicine*, **17**(8), 457–60.

Atkinson, P. (1979) *Research Design: Block 3B (Ethnography)*. Open University, Milton Keynes.

Bell, C. & Roberts, H. (1984) *Social Researching: Politics, Problem and Practice*. Routledge & Kegan Paul, London.

Brearley, S. (1990) *Patient Participation: the Literature*. Scutari Press, London.

Bryant, C. & Jary, D. (1991) *Giddens' Theory of Structuration: A Critical Appreciation*. Routledge, London.

Burrows, A. (1983) Patient-centred nursing care in a multi-racial society: the relevance of ethnographic perspectives in nursing curricula. *Journal of Advanced Nursing*, **8**(6), 477–85.

Bury, M. (1986) Social constructionism and the development of medical sociology. *Sociology of Health and Illness*, **8**, 137–69.

Bury, M. (1988) Meanings at risk: the experience of arthritis. In: *Living with Chronic Illness: the Experience of Patients and Their Families* (eds M. Bury, R. Anderson). Allen & Unwin, London.

Cornwell, J. (1984) *Hard Earned Lives: Accounts of Health and Illness from East London*. Tavistock, London.

Dobson, S. (1986) Ethnography: a tool for learning. *Nurse Education Today*, **6**, 76–9.

Doyal, L. (1993) On discovering the nature of knowledge in a world of relationships. In: *Nursing Art & Science* (ed. A. Kitson). Chapman & Hall, London.

Ersser, S. (1991) A search for the therapeutic dimensions of nurse–patient interaction. In: *Nursing as Therapy* (eds R. McMahon & A. Pearson). Chapman & Hall, London.

Ersser, S. (1995) *An ethnography of the therapeutic effect of nursing*. Unpublished PhD thesis, King's College, London.

Ersser, S. & Tutton, E. (1991) *Primary Nursing in Perspective*. Scutari Press, Harrow.

Fay, B. (1975) *Social Theory and Political Practice: Controversies in Sociology*. George Allen & Unwin, London.

Fetterman, D.M. (1989) *Ethnography Step by Step*. Applied Social Research Methods series, vol. 17. Sage, London.

Fitzpatrick, R. & Hopkins, A. (1983) Problems in the conceptual framework of patient satisfaction research: an empirical exploration. *Sociology of Health and Illness*, **5**(3), 297–311.

Foucault, M. (1986) Afterword: the subject and power. In: *Beyond Structuralism and Hermeneutics*. (H. Dreyfus & P. Rainbow). Harvester, Brighton.

Germain, C. (1979) *The Cancer Unit: An Ethnography*. Nursing Resources Inc., Wakefield, Massachusetts.

Germain, C. (1986) Ethnography: the method. In: *Nursing Research and Qualitative Perspective*. (eds P. Munhall & M. Oiler). Appleton-Century-Crofts, Norwich.

Glaser, B. (1978) *Theoretical Sensitivity*. The Sociology Press, San Francisco.

Hammersley, M. (1992) *What's Wrong with Ethnography? Methodological Explorations*. Routledge, London.

Hammersley, M. & Atkinson, P. (1983) *Ethnography: Principles in Practice*. Tavistock, London.

Lawler, J. (1991) *Behind the Screens: Nursing, Somology and the Problem of the Body*. Churchill Livingston, Melbourne.

May, C. (1992) Individual Care? Power and Subjectivity in Therapeutic Relationships. *Sociology* **26**(4), 589–602.

Morse, J. (1991) (ed.) *Qualitative Nursing Research: A Contemporary Dialogue*. Sage Publications, London.

Newby H. (1977) In the field: reflection on the study of Suffolk farmers. In: *Doing Sociological Research* (eds C. Bell & H. Newby). Allen & Unwin, London.

Ragucci, A.T. (1972) The ethnographic approach and nursing research. *Nursing Research*, **21**(6), 485–90.

Spradley, J.P. (1979) *The Ethnographic Interview*. Holt, Rinehart & Winston, New York.

Strong, P. & Robinson, J. (1988) *New Model Management: Griffiths and the NHS*. Nursing Policy Studies 3. Nursing Policy Studies Centre, University of Warwick, Coventry.

Waterworth, S. & Luker, K. (1990) Reluctant collaborators: do patients want to be involved in patient care? *Journal of Advanced Nursing*, **15**(8), 971–6.

Wax, R. (1971) *Doing Fieldwork: Warnings and Advice*. University of Chicago Press, Chicago.

Commentary on Chapter 4

Ray Fitzpatrick

A wide range of research strategies is needed to tease out the processes and outcomes of patient-centred care. Ethnographic methods have a long and distinguished history in the social sciences, especially in sociology and anthropology, and should provide health professionals with a rich and diverse range of insights into patient-centred care to complement the evidence provided by more quantitative methods. In particular it is clear from the examples provided in Chapters 4 and 12 by Steven Ersser and Angie Titchen, that ethnographic methods provide evidence that is graphic and vivid. At the heart of ethnography is the story, and readers are invited to follow the narrative of the ethnographer. One is able to enter the world or experiences of subjects who are studied by ethnographers in a way that no multivariate analysis in survey research or psychometric precision ever allows. Since many of our concerns in patient-centred care revolve around this task of empathy and understanding, this method deserves the closest attention.

It is worthwhile distinguishing some of the different ways in which ethnographic methods have illuminated patients' experiences. First, they have uncovered much of the hidden reality of how individuals with illness carry on their lives (Anderson & Bury 1988). We are made more aware of the diverse cognitive, emotional and practical demands imposed on patients as they cope with health problems. Ethnography can reveal unexpected features of patient-centred care. Thus in some circumstances patient-centred methods of history taking, which emphasize how the patient feels about his or her problem, may actually have unanticipated consequences of inhibiting the patient or inveigling him or her into undesired options (Silverman 1987).

Second, the story provided by ethnography can delineate the logic and meanings that underpin patients' statements and behaviours. Thus patients in consumer satisfaction surveys often complain about not being properly listened to by health professionals. The solution frequently proposed in the light of such evidence – interpersonal skills training – may convey the impression that politeness and good manners are the essence of patient-oriented care. In ethnographic studies it becomes clear that patients' complaints often reflect much more fundamental problems arising from lack of opportunity to discuss major concerns in relation to health problems (Fitzpatrick & Hopkins 1983).

Through Ersser's work we are forcibly reminded of how sensitive, subtle and specific are patients' observations of the health care that they receive. There may be a danger of making health professionals too self-conscious by feeding back to them the kind of evidence presented here of how their every gesture and action may be noted and interpreted by the patient. Instead we should be using such ethnographic evidence to delineate more clearly the various functions that can be carried out by health professionals. These affective functions are often achieved by the simplest of actions, for example by being present with the patient, and may therefore sometimes be unconscious.

The list would be long and diverse and the following only begins to address the potential functions of patient-centred care: making the patient more informed or in control, and providing reassurance, support, comfort, acceptance, legitimacy, confidence or optimism. The social sciences have not been particularly good in taking forward our language to delineate such affective functions, but are beginning to discover a framework for the analysis of caring in recent work on the sociology of the family (Finch & Grove 1983).

Ersser also invited the nurses in his study to reflect on their role and impact upon patients. This is invaluable. It is essential to be reminded that nurses, doctors and other health professionals have to strive for patient-centred care within their own personal limitations. There is substantial evidence of the different ways in which health professionals experience difficulties with patients with particular characteristics or problems. Patients may be viewed as 'good' or 'bad' depending on other perceptions such as whether they are 'responsible', 'uncomplaining' or 'not to blame' for their health problems (Dingwall & Murray 1983). Similarly time-pressures and the conflicting obligations that health professionals experience have been delineated in ethnographic research (Horobin & McIntosh 1983).

We need more thought to be given to the idea that nurses, doctors and other health professionals fulfil important roles in providing affective care, and that, as with any other scarce health care resource, there is therefore a continual problem of resource allocation by every health professional in the provision of caring. Social scientific research tends to emphasize the emergence of routines and 'rules of thumb' by health care providers to cope with such uncertainties and to make work more manageable. However, studies reported in this volume make it quite clear that there remains considerable discretion in how caring- functions under time constraints are carried out, and ethnographic work has a greater role to play in delineating this area of health professionals' decision-making.

Others have emphasized the value of the story as an aid to focusing us more clearly on the patient's experience (Charon 1989). It should be added that the social scientific, as opposed to literary, philosophical or other use of narrative, is distinctive. There are special responsibilities in relation to evidence, analysis and explanation. The evidence has to be as accurate as possible so that narratives maximally correspond to the settings described. This is not easy, given that in the health care context our narratives are drawn from patients and providers who themselves provide different accounts from each other (Eisenberg 1977; Sprangers & Aaronson 1992). The analysis, as well as being vivid and involving, has also to attempt to detach personal biases and follow canons of logic rather than the aesthetics of a good story. In the end the purpose of a social scientific story is an explanation of how things are the way they are.

Such explanations are still essential in the field of patient-centred care. We are only beginning to obtain systematic insights into how the processes of care relate to outcomes of value to patients. Especially with regard to caring, the complexities of delineating processes and outcomes are particularly daunting and we are in need of the help that good ethnography can give us.

References

Anderson, R. & Bury, M. (1988) *Living With Chronic Illness*. Unwin Hyman, London.

Charon, R. (1989) To listen, to recognize. In: *Perspectives in Medical Sociology* (ed. P. Brown) (ed. P. Brown), pp. 529–36. Wadsworth, California.

Dingwall, R. & Murray, T. (1983) Categorisation in accident departments: 'good' patients, 'bad' patients and 'children'. *Sociology of Health and Illness*, **5**, 127–48.

Eisenberg, L. (1977) Disease and illness: distinctions between professional and popular ideas of sickness. *Culture, Medicine and Psychiatry*, 1, 9–23.

Finch, J. & Grove, D. (eds) (1983) *A Labour of Love: Women, Work and Caring*. Routledge London.

Fitzpatrick, R. & Hopkins, A. (1983) Problems in the conceptual framework of patient satisfaction research: an empirical exploration. *Sociology of Health and Illness*, **5**, 297–311.

Horobin, G. & McIntosh, J. (1983) Time, risk and routine in general practice. *Sociology of Health and Illness*, **5**, 312–31.

Silverman, D. (1987) *Communication and Medical Practice*. Sage Publications, London.

Sprangers, M. & Aaronson, N. (1992) The role of health care providers and significant others in evaluating the quality of life of patients with chronic disease: a review. *Journal of Clinical Epidemiology*, **45**, 743–60.

5 ◆ Patient Representation: A Patient-Centred Approach to the Provision of Health Services

Ruth Ravich and Lucy Schmolka

Medical centres offer an impressive array of technology and services devoted to achieving state-of-the-art, skilfully delivered health care. Their size and complexity, however, create an impersonal, fragmented and mechanical environment which is often intimidating to patients and their families. Staff members, taxed by the demands of complicated technologies, financial constraints, government regulation and managerial and administrative duties, have become more function-oriented than patient-oriented, and individualized attention may be sacrificed. In order to deal with the challenges presented by an increasingly dehumanizing system, health care providers must focus on patient-centred care, guided by a realistic assessment of patients' needs.

To provide this focus, health care institutions in the USA have appointed patient representatives as an interface between the providers and the users of medical care. That this interface is essential is well documented in the literature. Szasz (1974) states that:

'It is not enough that we in the health professions do a technically competent job of healing the patient's body. We must do an equally competent job of safeguarding his dignity and self-esteem.'

Kosnik (1974) says that the health system must 'become responsive to the total needs of the patient ... familial, personal and societal'. One survey of outpatient and emergency departments (Dimensions in Health Services 1974) showed that 'the outstanding finding was the depersonalization shared by all patients who felt they were merely numbers, no longer individuals'.

Dissatisfaction with the delivery of medical care began to surface in the USA in the 1960s. One major factor was the focus on scientific rather than people-oriented medical education, which began in the early 1900s. At that time, medical school selection processes and curricula started to emphasize the sciences and downplay the art of medicine, limiting the capacity of many graduates to cope with the human concerns of patients and families. Ravich (1986) states that doctors who, in addition to treating illness, had traditionally been seen as counsellors and friends, were now often less able to establish good relationships with their patients.

Advances in medical technology provided another source of patient alienation. The increasing number of tests available to physicians all too often substituted for touching the patient, listening to his or her account of symptoms and problems and 'hearing' the latent content. Technologies led to physician specialization and increased emphasis on the treatment of specific organs, body parts or diseases instead of the 'whole' patient and his or her psychosocial as well as physical needs.

By the 1960s there were few family doctors or general practitioners who could be relied upon to provide patients with comprehensive information about their care and an explanation of hospital procedures. Rehr (1981) states that 'the binding ties between physicians and patients have been weakened and in some socioeconomic groups have been virtually destroyed'.

Ravich (1986) points out that advances in technology also led to specialization in other health care professions, among them nursing, physiotherapy, respiratory therapy and nuclear medicine. By the 1960s, professional staff working in large medical centres were divided into as many as 250 job classifications in 50 different occupational groups. Today's large medical centres employ staff in over 1000 different job categories, exposing patients and their families to as many as 65 different care givers on a single day, at a time when they are most vulnerable.

The media's attention to health care issues introduced other problems. Presentations, both fact and fiction, raised unrealistic expectations about the medical profession's ability to cure. At the same time, a growing emphasis on malpractice and mismanaged clinical care made patients fearful, even dissuading some from seeking timely medical intervention.

The creation of patient representative departments and the introduction of a Patient's Bill of Rights were efforts by the health care industry to reverse these unfavourable trends.

Patient representatives

In the 1960s there were no provisions within hospitals to mediate, advocate and educate patients to cope with the complex system, and no one to bring patients' perceptions of care to the attention of staff and administration. The patient advocacy concept, pioneered at The Mount Sinai Hospital in New York City, is the model for patient representation throughout the USA and abroad. The department was organized in 1966 to facilitate access to health care for community residents and to provide information, consultation, referral and advocacy services. Patient representatives were expected to intervene on behalf of patients who fell between the cracks of the hospital system, to identify recurring problems and to suggest solutions when these interfered with the delivery of comprehensive medical and social services.

Today, patient representatives, sometimes called health advocates or ombudsmen, have become an important bridge between providers and consumers of health care. They are generalists who address themselves to humanizing and personalizing the experience of patients and families in the overly specialized medical field. Their broad view of the organizations in which they serve places them in a position to recommend changes in policies and procedures to make these institutions more responsive to patient needs.

Patient representation is based on early forms of consumer advocacy. The ombudsman, 'one who acts on behalf of another', traditionally deals with a complex governmental bureaucracy, providing redress for individuals who encounter problems within institutions. A person acting as ombudsman is mentioned in the papers of the Ming Dynasty in China as early as the 14th century. The position was filled by an appointee of the emperor to protect the people against his advisors and tax collectors, who were usually his relatives. The Swedish governmental ombudsman, appointed by the parliament and reporting to it, was one of the models used in the development of the patient representative role (Reuss & Anderson 1966).

Unlike the Swedish and the British ombudsman (Rowat 1965), however, who are consulted only after other recourse is exhausted, patient representatives seek out patients in need of help or special attention as soon as possible after problems have surfaced, usually while they are still in the institution. This allows complaints to be dealt with and problems resolved before they escalate and become intractable. The governmental leverage of the ombudsman is not available to the patient representative, who must rely on knowledge of the functioning of the organization, on the ability to build co-operative relationships with all levels of staff and on administrative support.

Another model originally used to define patient representative services was the USA system of justice, which provides each side with a zealous advocate and in which opposing interests are expected to advance the work of the court. In contrast, however, patient representatives seek to resolve problems in a collegial rather than an adversarial manner.

A third model for the patient representation role, the Citizen Advice Bureau, is described by Kahn (1966). These Bureaux were organized in Great Britain during World War II to provide information and referral services to residents who were distressed or dislodged by the bombings. Similar services are provided by patient representatives who are knowledgeable about the health care system and resources within their institutions and communities.

Functions

Patient representatives are essentially problem solvers – for individuals, for departments and for systems. On a daily basis they expedite the resolution of the myriad difficulties that people encounter in any complex institution. The matters with which they deal range from diet to dying, from conflict arising from a breakdown in communications to major organizational flaws. They interpret policies and procedures to patients, families and visitors, help to guide them through the elaborate maze of the hospital world and bridge the inevitable gaps within the system. They provide information about patients' rights and assure that these are respected. They assist patients to become active participants in their care and they act as liaison among patients, families and staff when disagreements or potentially litigious situations arise. They support staff by intervening in response to difficult and complicated patient/family problems and concerns.

Resolutions range from a room change for a patient who is unhappy with a room-mate to calling a physician who, according to an irate patient or family, has not seen the patient for several days or has not provided sufficient information.

Example 1

Mr G.'s wife was very distressed because she felt that she was not receiving adequate answers to questions about her husband's condition. The patient representative found that Mr G. was being seen by a cardiac specialist, a vascular surgeon and a geriatrician, none of whom felt they were in charge of the case. A meeting with all three doctors and Mrs G. gave her the answers she needed, and all agreed that the geriatrician would be the contact physician for future information. In addition, because the patient representative also attended the meeting, she was able to reinforce the information when Mrs G. again became upset.

Example 2

Mrs T. was told by her surgeon that she would be receiving radiation therapy. She was under the impression that it would begin immediately and was distraught when she found she would have to wait five days. No one had explained that stimulation procedures had to be completed before therapy began. When these were explained, Mrs T. became less anxious.

If the patient's health care team – doctors, nurses, social workers – makes decisions with which the patient/family disagree, that disagreement may stem from a misunderstanding of the team's rationale, or may be because no one has elicited the patient's perception of his/her needs and abilities to carry out instructions. In these cases the patient representative might reconvene the 'team' to more fully explore the problems. In some situations a rigid protocol may need to be applied more flexibly (Ravich & Schmolka 1993).

Example 3

One case concerned a maternity patient who wanted her six-year-old daughter to visit her and to see the baby. Because the only person who could be asked to bring the daughter to the hospital was not available during regular sibling visiting hours, the patient representative arranged for the child to be allowed to visit at another time.

Patient representatives – who operate across medical, paramedical and nonmedical lines and deal with most services and all levels of personnel – provide a centralized, visible and efficient in-house mechanism for airing and addressing patient/family concerns and complaints. Their availability reduces the number of staff members to whom patients must explain problems and complaints and allows other staff to concentrate on their primary assignments. The representatives' overview of the institution allows them to serve as a highly sensitive thermostat, assessing the climate that pervades the institution and alerting administration to 'hot spots' that indicate patient and staff discontent (Ravich *et al.* 1969).

Although institutionally sponsored, patient representatives are expected to act as gadflies on the directors and managers of medical, paramedical and administrative services. They provide a consistent focus on patient perceptions of care, recurrent complaints and problem areas, recommending changes in hospital systems to facilitate patient-centred care (Ravich *et al.* 1969).

Issues addressed by patient representative departments include poor staff attitudes, inadequate communication, protest of discharge, confidentiality, informed consent, delay in treatment, institutional liability, refusal of treatment, release of medical information, lost items and dietary and housekeeping services.

Example 4

Ms P., a patient with irritable bowel syndrome was, according to the physician's notes, paranoid. She complained that the nurses were not washing their hands before caring for her. The patient representative asked the nursing supervisor to post a notice in the patient's room requesting all nursing personnel to wash their hands, to relieve her anxiety.

Example 5

Mr M. was protesting against his discharge because he did not feel well enough to go home. The patient representative found that home care was not in place and some test results had not been evaluated. When the physician was made aware of the problems, discharge was postponed. On the other hand, in the case of Mrs Q., the patient representative consulted with the physician who felt that discharge was appropriate. The patient was informed of the formal appeals mechanism that is available and how to initiate the process.

Example 6

Mr R.'s clothing and personal wheelchair could not be located when he was ready for discharge. It was found that, as he had been incompetent when he was admitted via the emergency department, he could not have cared for his possessions. Therefore the patient representative recommended that the hospital assume liability for their replacement. In another case, Mrs K. stated that she had removed her dentures, placed them on the bed and they had been removed with the bed linen. The laundry was contacted and the dentures located. If they had not been, however, the patient representative would have explained to Mrs K. that, as she was capable of taking care of her belongings, the hospital would not have been responsible for replacing them.

As a means of continuous quality improvement, recurrent problems, system gaps and areas of unresponsiveness to patients and families are pinpointed, investigated and analysed. A computer program specific to the Mount Sinai Hospital patient representative department permits monthly trending of patient problems and complaints by department, area and nursing unit. Given the approximately 16 000 cases dealt with annually, detailed documentation of complaints, problems and areas of unmet needs provides critical feedback to administrators. Recommendations for changes in policies and procedures and for staff training based on patient needs and perceptions are included in these reports, which provide a persuasive means of advocating systems change (Ravich & Schmolka 1993).

Example 7

Members of Ms B.'s family complained that they had waited in her room while she was in surgery. After several hours, they left to go to the cafeteria. They were therefore not on the nursing unit when the doctor called to inform them that the surgery had been completed. When they returned, the nursing shift had changed and the family did not receive information about the patient for several hours. The patient representative found that many families were having the same anxiety-provoking experience. Her recommendation, to locate a waiting area near the operating suite, was accepted. This facility allows surgeons to speak to the family as soon as the procedure is completed. An attendant has been engaged to maintain contact with the operating room, providing updates to the family regarding scheduling delays as well as completion of surgery and transfer of the patient to the recovery room.

Example 8

In 1967, when requests for interpreters to help staff communicate with non English-speaking patients were evaluated, it was found that medical information of a highly personal nature was often being translated by children or strangers. A notice in the hospital newspaper elicited response from 37 staff members who were fluent in 15 different languages and were willing to act as interpreters. This service has now been expanded to over 290 employees fluent in 60 languages.

Example 9

Patients who were to be hospitalized were receiving inappropriate or incomplete information about admitting procedures from their physicians. The patient representative and human resources departments arranged a series of programs for physicians' office staffs to inform them about hospital systems and introduce them to hospital personnel. This enabled them to present a realistic picture of the hospital experience to their patients.

In order to help all hospital staff focus on creating a patient-centred environment, patient representatives participate in orientation programmes for new employees and conduct frequent in-service staff training sessions. Subjects include patients' rights, advance directives (Appendix 5.1) and special services for patients with disabilities (Appendix 5.2). The representatives use patients' statements about the experiences of hospitalization and illness to demonstrate the need for sensitivity to the anxieties these engender. They also stress the importance of considering patient perceptions of care, whether or not these are factually accurate.

As advocates, patient representatives play a major role in the protection of patients' rights. In 1973 the American Hospital Association formulated a Patient's Bill of Rights (American Hospital Association 1973), which it disseminated to member institutions with the suggestion that it be given to all patients. Distribution of a patient's bill of rights is now mandated by individual states and by the Joint Commission for Accreditation of Health Care Organizations (JCAHO 1994). The Federal Government has also defined rights of patients and others: Americans With Disabilities Act 1991 (Appendix 5.1 in this chapter) and Federal Patient Self-Determination Act 1990 (Appendix 5.2). The latter mandates that each state establish a legal means to allow patients to express their wishes regarding treatment decisions in the event that they lose capacity to decide for themselves.

Two examples follow of cases that relate to the Self-Determination Act.

Example 10

Mr S., a young man with AIDS, had appointed his partner as his agent under the health care proxy law and had informed him that, in case he became terminally ill with no hope of recovery, he did not want to be placed on a respirator. However, when the time arrived, the man's mother insisted that she wanted every possible intervention to be utilized. The agent was intimidated by the mother's pressures and was not able to insist forcefully that the patient's wishes be fulfilled. A meeting arranged with several members of the family, the agent and the patient representative encouraged all to express their feelings and helped the mother to accept the patient's wishes to be allowed to die without being subjected to unwanted interventions.

Example 11

A nurse brought Mrs D.'s problem to the attention of the patient representative. The patient, a 93-year-old woman without capacity, had appointed her sister as her agent. The sister stated that Mrs D.'s expressed wish was to die with dignity and not to undergo any heroic measures. The physician, however, referred to a living will which was also in the chart. This document stated that heroic measures were to be withheld if the patient was in a 'terminal condition'. The physician told the patient representative that, as the patient had a one in 99 chance to improve after the treatment he was suggesting, he did not consider her condition terminal. He had therefore ordered a surgical procedure. In this case the proxy law, which supersedes the living will in New York State, was reviewed with the physician, who was then comfortable with the agent's decision to withhold further treatment.

The Americans with Disabilities Act mentioned above mandates 'nondiscrimination on the basis of disability in state and local government services'. Requirements include a provision that the disabled be afforded equally accessible and effective communication as that provided for other patients (Federal Register 1991). In many institutions the patient representative department is responsible for the provision of services to enable compliance with this law.

Patient representatives are also active in establishing and participating in ethics committees, which consider unresolved conflicts regarding issues such as initiating or discontinuing life support, refusing treatment, and disclosure of confidential information. In many facilities they also provide education in medical ethics and discuss policies and procedures regarding ethical issues that may be considered for adoption by the institution.

Research projects geared toward improving patient care and protection of patient's rights are being designed and carried out by patient representatives on an ongoing basis. One of these (Gauld-Jaeger 1990) focuses on matching patient and physician perceptions of readiness for discharge. Another attempts to monitor the effectiveness of the complaint management process (Rust 1992). Others evaluate the effectiveness of educational methods in encouraging people to appoint an agent who may decide about medical interventions the patient would want initiated or withheld in the event that he/she is unable to do so.

Additional patient representative functions include:

- advocacy for improved health care access;
- education for community residents regarding patients' rights and advance directives;
- liaison with the hospital community;
- linkage of elderly patients who are about to be discharged from the hospital with home care and telephone reassurance programs (AHA 1974).

As stated by the National Society for Patient Representation and Consumer Affairs (1995), the patient representative concept does not begin or end in the inpatient setting. Accommodating consumer needs and measuring consumer satisfaction is equally important for health maintenance organizations, ambulatory care clinics, home health agencies, physician group practices, nursing homes, and public health departments. Patient representatives answering to a variety of titles are working in every one of these settings.

Group practices and private medical partnerships use patient investigators or counsellors to screen inquiries, channel patients through the system, and respond to questions. As of now, most of these services are preventive in nature rather than part of a quality monitoring system.

The Society of Patient Representatives

Patient representation is unique in that its major *raison d'être* is to look at the health care experience from the patient's point of view. In 1969 a seminar sponsored by the training and research division of the United Hospital Fund of New York explored the possibilities of extending patient representative services. As an outcome, the Association of Patient Service Representatives was organized. In 1971 the American Hospital Association (AHA) accepted this Association as the Society of Patient Representatives of the AHA. Its aim, to promote the work of patient representatives, reflected the AHA's concern for helping its member institutions bring greater understanding of hospitals to consumers. It was anticipated that the Society would also act as a conduit to bring consumer concerns and needs to the attention of the health care industry.

Some patient representatives believed that this acceptance of the infant association by the AHA was a strategy for control of a group that might otherwise act in an adversarial role vis-à-vis its member hospitals (Ravich 1974). The umbrella of the AHA, however, enhanced the status of the field and promoted its expansion.

The place of a patient representative department in the institutional hierarchy has been a source of debate since the discipline was established. Most department administrators report to top or second-level administration and some are associate or assistant directors of their institutions. To be effective, however, representatives must be able to distance themselves from the problems and priorities of management (budget, space, staff demands) and focus attention on patient needs. This distancing, which is essential to the change agent role, may be difficult if the representatives are an integral component of the administrative group. On the other hand, being positioned as a decision maker may make it easier to effect broad-based change in institutional policies and procedures.

Just as early acceptance of this new field by the AHA was seen by some as a means of preventing challenge from outside the health care organization, so acceptance as part of the management team may be an attempt (conscious or unconscious) by an institution to co-opt its patient representatives. This concern is surfacing as some representatives become active members of hospital 'risk management' teams. While improving the climate of the institution and facilitating interpersonal and interdepartmental communications assists patients as well as risk management efforts, investigation of incidents and negotiation with patients on behalf of the institution may shift the focus from protecting the patient to protecting the facility.

Some community groups still voice concern about the ability of an advocate appointed by and responsible to the health care institution to effectively represent the patient. The Society points out that as they are members of the institution's staff and have a broad knowledge of the institution, its staff and its formal and informal rules systems, they are in the best position to communicate with other staff, to investigate, deal with and resolve problems as they occur rather than after the fact, and to negotiate for improved services. Ravich (1974) points out, however, that confrontation by organized groups outside the institution may be the only way to push toward significant reforms in the health delivery system.

Professional education

Since its organization, the Society of Patient Representatives, now known as the National Society for Patient Representation and Consumer Affairs of the American Hospital Association, has presented conferences and workshops to upgrade the knowledge and skills of its members. These have reflected the expanding roles of the membership as well as developing trends in health care delivery. Sessions have covered patients' rights and effective grievance mechanisms; ethical issues such as death and dying and assisted suicide; legal issues concerning patient representative responsibilities and risk management; and topics such as child abuse and rape crisis intervention. As many practitioners assumed administrative functions, sessions began to include management skills, long-range planning, quality assurance, budgeting, cost benefit and cost containment, and the re-engineering process.

Answering the need for a broad interdisciplinary education to prepare future leaders in this complex field, a Masters programme in health advocacy was established at Sarah Lawrence College in Bronxville, New York. Programme proposals were submitted in 1979, an interdisciplinary advisory committee was appointed and the first students matriculated in the autumn of 1980. The curriculum is based on biomedical sciences, health economics, health law, health care organization, ethical aspects of illness and medical treatment, health promotion and advocacy. Course work is conducted in seminars and tutorials with emphasis on student participation, library research and field work. Three 200-hour field placements with on-site supervised training is required. These enable students to apply classroom theory to practice and to develop their individual advocacy styles (Sarah Lawrence 1994) (Appendix 5.3 in this chapter).

Conclusions

Patient representatives facilitate education, communication and co-operation toward the overall institutional goal of promoting a positive consumer/provider relationship based on patient-centred care. Operating within the dual perspective of institution and consumer, patient representatives are important cogs in overall continuous quality assessment and improvement. They provide direct information and support for individual patients and their families. They help the institution respond effectively to complaints registered with governmental agencies. They track, trend and analyse recurrent system problems and, by working with administration, effect appropriate changes. They provide linkages among the various components of the system and between the institution and its target populations. They identify unmet needs and suggest innovative programs to attract and accommodate various potential patient populations.

Finally, the presence of a patient representative department makes a definitive statement to patients, their families, community agencies and medical centre staff that management is patient-oriented; it is concerned, willing to listen and, where appropriate, willing to take action to resolve problems, conflicts and misunderstandings; and it is committed to improving the hospital experience both in fact and perception. A successful patient representative program plays a critical role in increasing the organization's overall responsiveness to patient interests and in reducing the sense of alienation often perceived in the modern medical centre environment (Ravich & Schmolka 1993).

Reading guide

Friedman, E. *Choices and Conflict, Explorations in Health Care Ethics.* American Hospital Publishing, Chicago.

Galanti, G. *Caring for Patients from Different Cultures.* University of Pennsylvania Press, Philadelphia.

Gerteis, M., Edgman-Levitan, S., Daley, J. & Delbanco, T.L. (1993) *Through The Patient's Eye: Understanding and Promoting Patient-Centered Care.* Jossey-Bass, San Francisco.

Howe, E.G. (ed) (1993) *Journal of Clinical Ethics,* **4**(1), 3. Frederick, Maryland.

Komros, H. & Moore, N. (1993) *Patient Focused Healing: Integrating Caring and Curing in Healthcare.* Jossey-Bass, San Francisco.

Meyers, P. & Nance, D. (1986) *The Upset Book – A Guide for Dealing with Upset People.* Academic Publications, Notre Dame, Indiana.

References

AHA (1973) *Patient's Bill of Rights.* American Hospital Association, Chicago.

AHA (1974) American Hospital Association innovative programs. *Society of Patient Representatives Bulletin,* **5**

Dimensions in Health Services (1974) *Humanizing Patient Care.* Dimensions in Ottawa.

Federal Register (1991) Part IV. United States Department of Justice Rules and Regulations, **56**(144), 35711.

Gauld-Jaeger, J.R. (1990) *A Real or Imagined Threat.* Vanderbilt Medical Center, Nashville.

Greco, P.J. (1991) The Patient Self-Determination Act and the future of advance directives. *Annals of Internal Medicine,* **115**, 639.

JCAHO (1994) *Accreditation Manual for Hospitals* Joint Commission for Accreditation of Healthcare Organizations, Oakbrook Terrace, Illinois.

Kahn, A.J. (1966) *Neighborhood Information Centers: A Study and Some Proposals.* Columbia University School of Social Work, New York.

Kosnik, Rev. A. (1974) *Developing a health medical–moral committee.* Hospital Progress, St. Louis.

National Society of Patient Representation and Consumer Affairs (1995) In: *The Name of the Patient: Consumer Advocacy in Health Care.* American Hospital Association, Chicago.

Omnibus Budget Reconciliation Act of 1990. US Public Law No. 101–508.

Ravich, R. (1974) The Society of Patient Representatives. In: *In the Patient's Interest* (eds H. Rehr & M. Mailick, 1981), p. 144. Prodist, New York.

Ravich, R. (1986) *Patient advocacy.* Advocacy in Health Care. Humana Press, Clifton, New Jersey.

Ravich, R. & Schmolka, L. (1993) Patient representation as a quality improvement tool. *Mount Sinai Journal of Medicine,* **60** (5), 374–8.

Ravich, R., Rehr, H. & Goodrich, C. (1969) *Ombudsman: A New Concept in Voluntary Hospital Services,* pp. 311–20. Human Services and Social Work Responsibility. National Association of Social Workers, New York.

Rehr, H. (1981) The Current Climate in Hospital Care. In: *In the Patient's Interest* Prodist, New York.

Reuss, H.S. & Anderson, S.V. (1966) The Ombudsman: Tribute of the People. *Annals of the American Academy of Political and Social Science,* **363**(1), 44.

Rowat, D.C. (1965) *The Ombudsman: Citizen's Defender.* Allen & Unwin, London.

Rust, T.R. (1992) *Monitoring Complaint Management Effectiveness.* Owen Graduate School of Management, Vanderbilt University, Nashville.

Sarah Lawrence (1994) *Catalog for Health Care Advocacy Program.* Sarah Lawrence College, Bronxville, New York.

Szasz, T. (1974) Illness and dignity. *Journal of the American Medical Association,* Chicago.

Appendix 5.1

The Federal Americans With Disabilities Act 1991 mandates that public institutions receiving federal funds provide the same services to all individuals, regardless of physical or mental disabilities.

Special services for patients with disabilities

At The Mount Sinai Medical Centre, the following aids are provided.

For the visually impaired:

- Large-type books and 'Talking Books' with earphones are available.
- An audio tape enumerates the Patient's Bill of Rights.
- The Patient's Bill of Rights is available in Braille.

For speech and hearing-impaired patients and those with language barriers:

- Communi-Card, for general use (Fig. 5.1), and Communi-Card 2, for emergency and special care units (Fig. 5.2), present easy-to-understand pictograms illustrating symptoms, needs (medical, physical and emotional), as well as health care professionals to whom a patient may want to speak. These enable patients to communicate with staff members of family by pointing to a need or responding by

Communi-Card

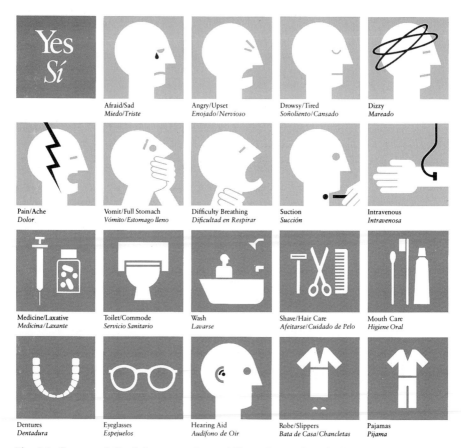

Yes
Sí

Afraid/Sad
Miedo/Triste

Angry/Upset
Enojado/Nervioso

Drowsy/Tired
Soñoliento/Cansado

Dizzy
Mareado

Pain/Ache
Dolor

Vomit/Full Stomach
Vómito/Estomago lleno

Difficulty Breathing
Dificultad en Respirar

Suction
Succión

Intravenous
Intravenosa

Medicine/Laxative
Medicina/Laxante

Toilet/Commode
Servicio Sanitario

Wash
Lavarse

Shave/Hair Care
Afeitarse/Cuidado de Pelo

Mouth Care
Higiene Oral

Dentures
Dentadura

Eyeglasses
Espejuelos

Hearing Aid
Audífono de Oir

Robe/Slippers
Bata de Casa/Chancletas

Pajamas
Pijama

Fig. 5.1 Communi-Card for general use. (*Above:* front of card. *Opposite:* reverse of card.)

a nod or blink to an indicated pictogram. The cards are presented in English and Spanish, and can be easily adapted to any language.
- Full-time Spanish-speaking patient representatives are on staff (to accommodate the Mount Sinai community population).
- 'Interpreteam' staff members are fluent in 60 languages.
- Conference calls in over 140 languages can be arranged through an AT&T (American Telephone and Telegraph Company) language line.

For the hearing disabled:

- Telephone amplifiers and telecommunication devices for the deaf (TDDs) are supplied.

This card has been prepared to assist you in communicating with your family, friends and hospital staff.

Estos dibujos se han preparados para que usted se pueda comunicar con su familia, sus amistades, y los empleados del hospital.

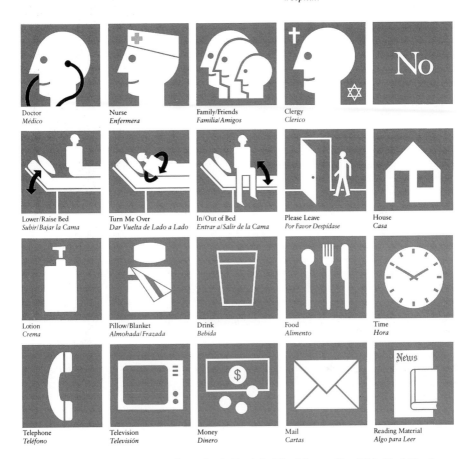

Doctor *Médico*	Nurse *Enfermera*	Family/Friends *Familia/Amigos*	Clergy *Clerico*	No
Lower/Raise Bed *Subir/Bajar la Cama*	Turn Me Over *Dar Vuelta de Lado a Lado*	In/Out of Bed *Entrar a/Salir de la Cama*	Please Leave *Por Favor Despídase*	House *Casa*
Lotion *Crema*	Pillow/Blanket *Almohada/Frazada*	Drink *Bebida*	Food *Alimento*	Time *Hora*
Telephone *Teléfono*	Television *Televisión*	Money *Dinero*	Mail *Cartas*	Reading Material *Algo para Leer*

(Reproduced with permission from Ruth Ravich, The Mount Sinai Medical Center, Patient Representative Department (original concept by Linda Marks.)

- Sign-language interpreters are available.
- The international symbol for the deaf, placed on bed and medical records, with the patient's permission, alerts staff to special communication needs.
- A video *Caring for the Hearing Impaired* is used for staff education.

Appendix 5.2

Advance directives

The Federal Patient Self-Determination Act (PSDA), (Omnibus Reconciliation Act of 1990), mandates that patients be informed about

Communi-Card **2**

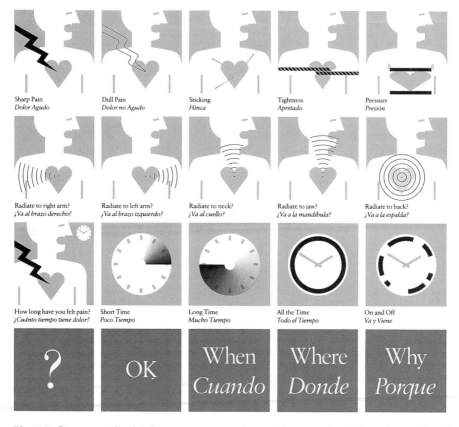

Sharp Pain *Dolor Agudo*	Dull Pain *Dolor no Agudo*	Sticking *Hinca*	Tightness *Apretado*	Pressure *Presión*
Radiate to right arm? *¿Va al brazo derecho?*	Radiate to left arm? *¿Va al brazo izquierdo?*	Radiate to neck? *¿Va al cuello?*	Radiate to jaw? *¿Va a la mandíbula?*	Radiate to back? *¿Va a la espalda?*
How long have you felt pain? *¿Cuánto tiempo tiene dolor?*	Short Time *Poco Tiempo*	Long Time *Mucho Tiempo*	All the Time *Todo el Tiempo*	On and Off *Va y Viene*
?	OK	When *Cuando*	Where *Donde*	Why *Porque*

Fig. 5.2 Communi-Card 2 for emergency and special care units. (*Above:* front of card. *Opposite:* reverse of card.)

and assisted in executing advance directives. Although the type of instrument adopted by individual states may vary, the intent is to assure that a person's wishes about medical treatment are carried out in the event that he/she becomes incapacitated and cannot make these decisions.

The PSDA requires institutions that receive federal funding for patient care to develop and maintain written policies and procedures that provide written information for adults to whom the institution provides care. This material must describe:

- an individual's rights under state law to make decisions about medical care, including the right to accept or refuse medical and surgical treatment.

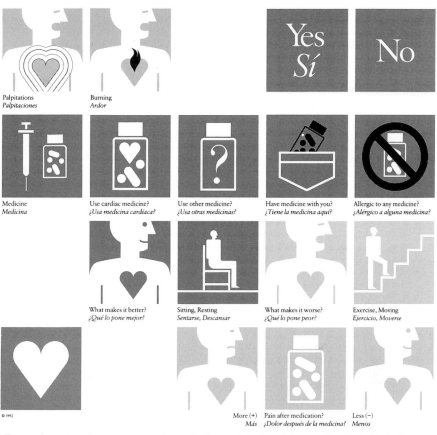

This card has been prepared to assist you in communicating with hospital staff in the emergency area and special care units.

Esta tarjeta ha sido preparada para ayudarle a comunicarse con el personal en la sala de emergencia y en la unidad de cuidado intensivo.

Palpitations
Palpitaciones

Burning
Ardor

Yes
Sí

No

Medicine
Medicina

Use cardiac medicine?
¿Usa medicina cardíaca?

Use other medicine?
¿Usa otras medicinas?

Have medicine with you?
¿Tiene la medicina aquí?

Allergic to any medicine?
¿Alérgico a alguna medicina?

What makes it better?
¿Qué lo pone mejor?

Sitting, Resting
Sentarse, Descansar

What makes it worse?
¿Qué lo pone peor?

Exercise, Moving
Ejercicio, Moverse

© 1992

More (+)
Más

Pain after medication?
¿Dolor después de la medicina?

Less (−)
Menos

(Reproduced with permission from Ruth Ravich, The Mount Sinai Medical Center, Patient Representative Department (original concept by Linda Marks.)

- an individual's rights under state law to formulate advance medical directives, such as a living will or durable power of attorney for health care, to guide the provision of care when the individual loses capacity;
- the policies and procedures that the institution has developed to honour these rights.

The types of advance directives most commonly used are the living will and the durable power of attorney for health care decisions or health care proxy. The living will enumerates the person's wishes concerning medical care decisions when the patient is judged to be terminally ill or permanently unconscious. The durable power of attorney for health care decisions, or proxy, allows a person to appoint an agent to make decisions in the event he/she is unable to do so, even temporarily.

The federal law does not override state laws that permit a health care provider to decline to comply with an advance directive as a matter of conscientious objection, as long as the patient has been informed about this aspect of the law.

The legislation also requires institutions to provide educational programmes on advance directives for their staff and communities.

Appendix 5.3

Master's programme in health advocacy, Sarah Lawrence College, Bronxville, New York. Joan Marks, Director.
Joan Marks and Ruth Ravich, Co-Founders, 1979–80; Co-Directors, 1980–85.

Course of study

Health advocacy 1 introduces the concepts, models and practice of advocacy. It emphasizes the roles which health advocates play in affecting health policy and service delivery. Analysis of organizations and communities provides an understanding of power and decision making. Strategies for increasing the impact of advocates on the health care system are explored.

Health advocacy 2 covers patient representation and the functions of patient advocates in hospitals and alternative health care facilities. Studies, in conjunction with hospital field work, emphasize patients' rights, grievance mechanisms and factors influencing access to and use of health care services.

Health advocacy 3 explores ethical dilemmas which confront clinicians, patients, families and administrators. It provides an ethical framework from which to consider treatment decisions. Issues that arise in ethical decision making when special populations are involved are discussed.

Health care history examines the component parts of the health care system: professionals, institutions, consumers, government policies and health-related industries.

Human anatomy and physiological systems enables students to understand biological concepts and medical terminology. It concentrates on normal human beings and introduces the effects of pathology on human health.

The nature of illness and caring provides an understanding of human suffering. Discussions focus on meeting the demands of the suffering person.

Evaluation and assessment: methods and issues uses scientific methods to evaluate health care programs. Basic research concepts and methods, including data analysis, are explored.

The economics of health explores the nature of economic analysis. It examines fundamental principles and their applications to policy development, resource allocation, program evaluation, insurance, regulation and reimbursement.

Health care from policy to practice: politics, organization and management provides a study of public and private forces in the health care system. Organization and management of various types of health care facilities are studied, as well as the financial and administrative supports required.

Health law covers basic health issues and problems that can be solved through legal means. Topics include locating legal information, corporate law as applied to health care institutions, regulation of health services, patients' rights, medical malpractice and legal problems relating to terminally ill and psychiatric patients.

Field training three 200-hour supervised field placements. On-site training in health care institutions and other areas of health advocacy allows the application of classroom theory to practice. Individual conferences explore aspects of the field experience.

Commentary on Chapter 5

Shirley McIver

The advances in medical technology and changes in medical education mentioned by Ravich and Schmolka in this chapter are not confined to the USA and so it is no surprise to find that patients in the UK have also complained about impersonal hospital care. Medical specialization may well be one of the reasons patients find their information and communication needs are not satisfied and why these issues are common problems occurring in the work of the health ombudsman and mentioned in surveys of patients' views.

The Patient's Charter has begun to focus attention on the psycho-social and information needs of patients and relatives by making it clear that patients have the right to be given a clear explanation of any treatment proposed, including any risks and any alternatives, before they decide whether they will agree to treatment; also to be given detailed information on local health services and to have care which respects privacy, dignity and religious and cultural beliefs. This means that health professionals are now increasingly under pressure to provide better information and a more personal service to patients.

It is highly likely that an innovation which has helped to increase the responsiveness of hospitals to patients' interests in the USA could have the same effect in this country. Indeed roles very similar to that of the patient representative have been developing in the UK since the late

1980s. Often called patient liaison officers or customer relations managers, they are usually employed to sort out patients' concerns and help provide them with information.

In 1992 the NHS Management Executive funded a project designed to look more systematically at the role of the patient representative in helping to make services less bureaucratic and more friendly to patients. It was set up as an action research project, under the management of the National Association of Health Authorities and Trusts (NAHAT). Two pilot sites at Brighton Health Care Trust and Frenchay Health Care Trust were partly funded for a year to employ a patient's representative. I was employed as a part-time researcher for two years to follow their experiences, set them within a wider context and disseminate information about the project. The experiences of the two pilot sites, and of those in similar posts, have been documented in two reports produced by NAHAT (McIver 1993, 1994).

UK pilot sites

In the UK, patients' representatives operate in a way similar to their colleagues across the Atlantic. This is not surprising because the blueprint for the role at the two pilot sites was based upon the USA model. They were given two main tasks:

(1) to respond directly to patients and relatives who feel their concerns are not being resolved in a satisfactory manner. In this way they deal with patients' issues quickly and prevent problems from escalating;
(2) to work with other staff to improve services so that they become more patient focused and so that problems experienced by patients are less likely to occur again.

There have been differences in the way the two pilot sites have developed; at Brighton, for example, Bec Hanley, the first patient's representative (called an advocate) was promoted to assistant director of quality and Penny Dunman was recruited to replace her, whilst at Frenchay, June Leat made a successful business case for an assistant to help her. But there have also been many similarities in their experiences.

Confusion over the responsibilities of the patients' representative was experienced initially at both sites, and they have clarified the role in a similar way by setting standards of work. They have also come to similar conclusions about the usefulness of computerized systems for recording and analysing their work, and linking it to formal complaints and untoward incidents.

Their impact on complaints received has also been similar and shows that providing an informal way for users to make comments and complaints does not significantly increase (or decrease) formal complaints. Their impact can be observed in other ways. Due to advice from the patients' representative, the clarity and focus of many formal complaints is improved, making them easier to handle. Also there is some evidence that the informal route picks up different types of concerns and problems from the formal. Issues concerning deceased patients, supplies and equipment, mixed sex wards and the complaints system, are examples recorded by June Leat at Frenchay.

The project was able to show that the patients' representatives at the pilot sites were able to improve things for many patients, helping both individuals with their concerns and also many more patients through their work with colleagues on issues raised by patients. However, the second report sounded a note of concern that patients' representatives were often seen as a way of 'plugging a gap' in the service to patients and this could leave them with a mammoth task unless they were part of a team of people working to improve services from the patients' point of view. It is interesting to note that Ravich and Schmolka refer to patient representative departments rather than to individuals working alone.

When the UK pilot project started, there were approximately eight similar posts in existence, but by the end of 1994 there were over 30 including all but one of the original posts. There is as yet no national society for patient representation, as there is in the USA, but the pilot project established a network which continues to hold regular meetings. The network has been invited by the Association for Quality in Healthcare (AQH) to become a special interest group of this national organization and so it is possible that this may serve a similar purpose.

The wider UK picture

At present the majority of patients' representatives are employed in the acute sector, but similar posts are beginning to occur in primary and community care where they are usually based around specific client groups. It is easy to see why this is the case because vulnerable people will need help across a range of services provided by different agencies. This is probably also why posts in these areas tend to be linked to the wider advocacy movement.

Advocacy posts in the health service are generally managed independently of the health care provider in order to lessen conflict of interest for the advocate. There have been exceptions – in particular the Linkworker posts established as a result of the Asian Mother and Baby Campaign. However, these posts, and many of the bilingual advocacy posts which have been set up to improve access to health services for black and minority ethnic people, have run into difficulties (Hicks & Hayes 1991). Other models, such as those managed by community health councils, may be more effective (Cornwell & Gordon 1984).

Ravich and Schmolka raise this issue, pointing out that community groups in the USA are still voicing concerns about the ability of an advocate appointed by and responsible to the health care institution to effectively represent patients. In common with the USA Society for Patient Representation and Consumer Affairs, the UK pilot project found that patients' representatives were in the best position to investigate, deal with and resolve problems as they occur rather than after the fact, and to work with other staff to improve services. The advocate and patient representative functions are complementary, with advocates being in a better position to work on behalf of vulnerable people across a wide range of health and social services.

It is likely that this dispute about 'whose side' the patients' representative is on will continue until research is carried out on the effectiveness of the different types of advocacy roles. Very few advocacy projects have been evaluated and until they are, it is unlikely that the concept will be taken seriously by health professionals. Unlike the USA, the UK has no training for patients' representatives and this may be an area which can be examined by the special interest group of the Association for Quality in Healthcare. Certainly there is a need for accredited training for both advocates and patient's representatives.

Despite these areas for development, patient representation in the UK is well on the road to becoming established in the way Ravich and Schmolka describe has occurred in the USA. This is likely to continue because it is being supported by the introduction of consumerism into the NHS, which has encouraged the reform of the complaints procedure, a focus on patients' rights, and a concern for patient empowerment.

References

Cornwell, J. & Gordon, P. (1984) *An Experiment in Advocacy: The Hackney Multi-Ethnic Women's Health Project.* King's Fund Centre, London.

Hicks, C. & Hayes, L. (1991) Linkworkers in antenatal care: facilitators of equal opportunities in health provision or salves for the management conscience? *Health Services Management Research,* **4**(2), 89–93.

McIver, S. (1993) *Investing in Patient's Representatives.* NAHAT, Birmingham.

McIver, S. (1994) *Establishing Patient's Representatives.* NAHAT, Birmingham.

6 ◆ The Named Nurse

Stephen Graham Wright

The named nurse, midwife and health visitor

> 'They were nothing more than people, by themselves. Even paired, any pairing, they would have been nothing more than people by themselves. But together, they have become the heart and muscles and mind of something perilous and new, something strange and giving and great. Together, all together, they are the instruments of change.' (Hulme 1986)

The term nurse is used throughout this chapter, for simplicity, to include midwives and health visitors.

The emergence of the named nurse concept

Emerging from government policy in 1990 was the concept of the Citizen's Charter. The expressed aim was to ensure that various public services would make explicit to those who use them what rights and standards of service could be expected. The intention was to create greater public awareness of what these services should be providing. By empowering people in this way it was felt that they would be better able to ensure that high quality services are achieved.

Individual health services began to publish their Patient's Charters and make them available, including the health services of England, Scotland, Northern Ireland and Wales (DoH 1992; NIHPSO 1992; Scottish Office 1991; Welsh Office 1991). Millions of the full versions of the charters were distributed, and summary papers were posted to every home.

The English charter (DoH 1992) states:

> 'The charter standard is that you should have a named, qualified nurse midwife or health visitor who will be responsible for your nursing or midwifery care.'

The Welsh Office document (1991) has similar wording, but does not indicate clearly if this is a 'right' or a 'standard'. The Northern Ireland charter is explicit that patients have a right to a named nurse (NIHPSO 1992). The Scottish Office charter (1991) makes no mention of the named nurse, although subsequent guidance has indicated that the named nurse should be implemented throughout Scotland by 1997.

Much debate has continued on the effectiveness of these charters.

Were they a glossy public relations exercise, but with no real benefits? Were they being used to cover up failings in the services? Were people really able to use them to assert their rights, and if so, was there any discernible effect on the service? The debate continues, and this chapter will seek to address some of these issues by focusing on one of the principal elements of the charters: the named nurse, midwife and health visitor concept.

One of the criticisms of the charters has been about their glossy production and presentation. They give the impression to the public that something new and exciting provided by the government is on offer. In reality, they often affirm what are existing rights and standards that are already enshrined in laws, policies, or generally accepted current practices (Cole & Davidson 1992). Robinson (1992) believed that their arrival at the time of a general election was not insignificant – encouraging people to feel that all was well with the NHS or perhaps encouraging nurses to vote in a particular way because something (i.e. the status of the named nurse) seemed to be on offer.

The assumption underpinning the named nurse approach is that better care is available if individual nurses can be responsible for the overall care of particular patients. Historically, nurses have organized care in many ways. It is beyond the scope of this chapter to explore these methods in detail, but a recent short paper (RCN 1992a) succinctly summarizes these. Broadly, they fall into two groups.

The first is work centred, where nurses are allocated to perform certain tasks in relation to patient care. Task allocation allots responsibility for carrying out delegated tasks to all patients; for example, doing all the dressings, the baths or the drug round – usually on the basis of a hierarchy of seniority among the nurses. The most junior nurse gets what are judged the most menial tasks, the most senior the more 'important' tasks such as organizing the doctor's round (Pearson & Vaughan 1986). Although this is often associated with hospital work, a similar approach can be found in community care as well. Thus, the approach focuses on organizing staff to ensure that a minimum standard of physical care is provided for all patients. Unfortunately, large areas of care may be omitted as they are often difficult to allocate, especially relating to the nature of the nurse–patient relationship and how nurses work with patients to help them 'feel' better (Henderson 1980).

The second approach encompasses patient-centred methods, such as team nursing or midwifery (where the care of a group of patients is allocated on a continuous basis to a group of nurses managed by a team leader), or a primary nurse (an individual nurse taking complete responsibility for the management of a patient's care).

A variety of methods such as these are used to allocate nurses to the overall care of patients and all are seen as options for implementing the named nurse (Wright 1993). In the case of primary nursing, this includes a particular nurse taking overall responsibility for the care of a patient or group of patients for the whole of the patient's stay in the relevant setting (Pearson, 1988; Wright 1990). Some methods have been long established; for example, it is rare for health visitors to organize care in any other way than their own 'case method' – a client caseload on a long-term basis.

The boundaries between these methods may often be blurred and there may be a lack of clarity among nurses about precisely which method they are using (NHSE 1994). However, all have the intent of identifying particular nurses with the responsibility for the care of particular patients. Even so, organizing care in such ways is no guarantee that care will be any more personal. Allocating the nurse to the patient will not necessarily, of itself, improve the quality of care unless other factors are in place.

The shift from task allocation to patient-centred methods over recent years has in part been driven by both patients and nurses as each has demanded improvements in the quality of care. There has been a desire to make care more humane and personal and to escape from the 'production line concept of care' (Briggs 1972; Pearson 1988). Recent surveys have supported the view that, over the past decade, the organization of nursing care has been in transition. Task allocation, the dominant method of organizing care in hospitals in the early 1980s (about 75% of settings in 1981) fell to about 10% in 1992. Primary nursing has moved from less than 1% to 16% in the same period, while over a third of other settings use either team nursing or patient allocation (usually a nurse looking after the same patients on a shift by shift basis) respectively (IMS 1992; Audit Commission 1991).

It has been suggested that reorganizing care is no guarantee that the quality of the nurse–patient relationship will improve. Furthermore, questions could be asked about the reliability of the data, given that nurses may sometimes have difficulty in defining which approach they are using. Even so, the figures do suggest that an enormous shift has taken place. This lends strength to the argument that nursing was already in transition before the charters were published. Named nursing, though it may not have been explicitly defined as such, was being deployed in a variety of settings using a variety of methods – and is increasingly being so. In this sense, the charters may be seen to have capitalized on a trend that was already under way, given it a more defined public profile and, perhaps, encouraged others to make a shift in order to meet charter requirements.

The charters, strictly speaking, apply only to the public sector, but clearly the independent sector is unlikely to allow itself to lag behind in something that the public sector provides. Meanwhile, purchasing or commissioning health authorities at local level are writing the national charter standards and rights into local contracts with trusts and other bodies (the providers). There is an added incentive at management level to ensure these rights and standards (including the named nurse) are delivered, because purchasers can take punitive measures of sanctions against trusts which fail to meet contractual requirements.

When the named nurse is included as a right, there is little scope for negotiation. A right has to be delivered. A standard offers some degree of flexibility; for example, if a purchaser agrees a contract with a trust, to include the named nurse, it may specify that the standard must be achieved, say, 80% of the time. Monitoring mechanisms will reveal if this is being achieved (NHSE 1994), with serious implications for both parties if it is not.

One survey suggests that in England, 95% of settings had been able to implement the named nurse standard (DoH 1994). However, this survey was very limited in its methods. A questionnaire was sent to all provider units, and included a question related to the implementation of the named nurse. When 95% respond positively, does this mean that the named nurse has been implemented across the board in a whole unit, or that it is happening in only one part of it?

Clearly there are major implications for nurses, midwives and health visitors as the national charter standards and rights are written into local contracts. In addition, the charters are in the public domain and will inevitably raise public expectation that a named nurse is always available to them (Higgins 1992). If the previously cited surveys are considered, it seems that most nurses are well on the way to implementing the named nurse standard and rights and were indeed doing so before the charters were published. The perception, therefore, that the concept is politically imposed from above seems overly simplistic. A more accurate view may be that a particular political perspective saw an opportunity to capitalize on something which nurses were already pursuing, and claimed the credit for it!

Alternatively, a less cynical view may be that the named nurse aspect of the charters was the product of genuine conviction that such an approach is good for patients and should therefore be acknowledged. Certainly it seems unlikely that its inclusion in a political initiative would have been possible without a considerable period of groundwork. Major professional organizations, such as the Royal College of Midwives and the Royal College of Nursing, had been lobbying for the central role of nursing to be recognized for some time. The former Chief Nurse, Dame Anne Poole, is believed to have included the named nurse concept in her targets on taking up her post in 1982. Meanwhile, the Patient's Charters were being produced at a time when considerable personal lobbying of ministers by nurses, including units in many sites where primary nursing had been implemented successfully, were taking place in the late 1980s.

It is clear, then, that a groundswell of change in the organization of patient care by nurses was already under way, before the Patient's Charters were published. The author's own personal experience is one of working with nurses at clinical level in a unit dedicated to making changes in nursing practice. This nursing development unit, as it became known, at Tameside General Hospital near Manchester, was one of the earliest such projects in the UK. Nurses there transformed care, including moving away from the ritualized approaches associated with task allocation, to the personalized values and practices inherent in primary nursing.

This clinical experience led the author into involvement in policy development work at national level, including work with the Royal College of Nursing and the Department of Health's Patient's Charter team in the early 1990s. This is one example among many of how nurses can bring their clinical knowledge and expertise to bear on wider health policy developments. Even so, it is perhaps most significant to recall that organizing care in named nurse ways is very much rooted in developments at clinical level. Many initiatives in nursing arise from academic circles or through management edict. In this case there is much evidence to support the view of named nursing as a largely practice-led phenomenon. It may subsequently have been taken up as a national cause, but it remains very much a movement with its roots in nursing practice.

Therefore the arrival of the named nurse in the Patient's Charters is probably not attributable to one cause. It has emerged, rather, from a number of factors which have come together at a particular time.

Practical and ethical implications

While the Patient's Charters and the explicit announcement of the named nurse may be innovations, these took place upon a groundswell of reorganizing and rethinking in nursing that appeared to gather pace in the 1980s. This movement for change in nursing – including an assertion of the value of nursing (and the roles of women especially), and an exploration of clinical innovation and research – has been seen by some as a distinct phenomenon. Salvage (1990) has coined the phrase 'new nursing' to encapsulate these notions. In this context, the named nurse may be seen as but one piece in a larger puzzle. The maturation of the discipline of nursing has reached a point where it is possible for a national standard or right of access to the service to be asserted. At the same time, the establishment of this approach itself feeds back into nursing to stimulate yet more change.

The publication of the charters may lead some to believe that the change to named nursing was being implemented from the top down. However, as we have seen, the process was already under way. In settings where the named nurse was not being practised, inevitably there has been pressure to make the change. In many respects this is counterproductive.

Approaches to change in nursing suggest tht 'bottom-up' methods which involve the staff at clinical level and ensure they have 'ownership' of this change process, are far more likely in the long term to be effective (Black 1993; Pearson 1992; Wright 1989). In some settings, it has been necessary for managers and others to step back from the pressure of the imperatives to reach targets and to give nurses at clinical levels the time and support to implement the changes successfully. The case studies provided in a Department of Health publication (Wright 1993) reinforce the view that a number of factors are critical to success, including:

(1) managerial and educational support and commitment to facilitate, not control, the change and provide resources;
(2) the provision of steering groups to guide the process at all organizational levels, including clinical staff;
(3) the presence of an effective clinical leader (e.g. team leader, charge nurse);
(4) a planned approach to change, including adequate time for implementation;
(5) beginning with pilot sites where there is staff willingness;
(6) time and support to build knowledge and skills amongst staff;
(7) building in an evaluation programme to monitor success;
(8) identifying responsibilities of each member of staff;
(9) the opportunity to try out different systems.

These principles appear to be common factors in those settings which have implemented the named nurse successfully.

Evaluation to monitor the degree of success has also taken many forms. A recent NHS Executive (1994) survey illustrates some of these varied approaches. A combination of factors is used in many settings, from informal observation through to rigorous standard setting and monitoring. Questionnaires, standards, interview schedules and so on, can provide some degree of information about the implementation of the named nurse. Their scope, however, is limited.

Asking questions, for example, which identify organizational aspects of the named nurse may give some indicators about successful implementation; for example, do all staff wear name badges? Is the named nurse identified on the care plan? Is the patient given a named nurse identification card? (NHSE 1994). It is much more problematic, for example, to identify how nurse and patient feel about each other, or whether the relationship is therapeutic. Very little rigorous research, as yet, has taken place in this respect, although some early work alludes to positive patient outcomes (Fanning 1993).

The benefits of the therapeutic relationships in nursing are well documented; for example, Carr Hill *et al.* (1992); Kitson (1988); Pearson *et al.* (1988); RCN (1992b). However, as has been suggested, reorganizing care to place individual responsibility for patients with individual nurses, is no guarantee that a therapeutic relationship will emerge, particularly if nurse–patient contact time is relatively small.

The often cited work of Menzies (1961) suggests that nurses used task allocation to protect themselves from the anxiety of involvement in a nurse–patient relationship. Yet the named nurse concept demands such a relationship if its purpose is to be realised. In the transition from impersonal methods, such as task allocation, to more personal methods, such as team nursing, it is clear that nurses need various methods of support, including:

- access to clinical supervision;
- good team relationships;
- a supportive management climate;
- opportunities for personal and professional growth (RCN 1992c; Wright 1990).

If old methods which appear, however dubiously, to have protected nurses in the past (for example, task allocation and hierarchical control) are removed, then clearly nurses need avenues of support to help them in their daily work. The nurse–patient relationship is inherently stressful, but this can be managed, and prevented from reaching pathological proportions, by effective management and supportive techniques (Snow & Willard 1989).

Partners in care?

The named nurse concept aims to bring greater clarification to the responsibilities of the nurse in the nurse–patient relationship. It also seeks to provide the patient with a focal point, in what can otherwise be a very confusing health care system. Pearson (1988) asserts that it is to nurses that patients look to humanize the system or, as Peplau (1952) states, to be their 'professional friend'. The common thread here is that the nurse is best placed to be the patient's principal guide through the complexities of health care. This notion is not without controversy.

Some doctors are hostile to the named nurse concept, because it is seen as an invasion by nurses of doctors' territory (Cole & Davidson 1992). Hugman (1991) believes that the issue of territory has very little to do with the quality of patient care; it is rather to do with the maintenance of traditional medically dominated power structures. Meanwhile, anecdotal evidence from other professions suggests that the question was often asked – if a named nurse, why not a named physiotherapist, dietician or speech therapist?

Some in leadership positions in nursing, especially those at ward sister, charge nurse or team leader level, are reported to have expressed fears that their role and purpose will be eroded if more responsibility for care is passed to others. The named nurse principle clearly indicates that the named nurses are direct care givers (Wright 1993), not necessarily giving all the care but being involved sufficiently to co-ordinate the work of others in their absence. It has been asserted that the named nurse concept will not develop where those in clinical leadership positions seek to use traditional methods of hierarchical control in the clinical area (NHSE 1994). This is not to say that these roles are no longer needed, rather that they need to emerge more as clinical consultants, monitoring, co-ordinating and supervising, as well as having a direct responsibility for some element of nursing practice (for example, by having a caseload, part caseload, or contributing as team members themselves). Indeed, there is strength in the argument that named nurses need this back-up as part of their overall support strategy if they are to survive in the complex world of the nurse–patient relationship.

The named nurse principle is underpinned by the concept of partnership between nurse and patient (Hancock 1992), as well as between nurses themselves and other health care workers. Yet it seems to be a partnership of unequals. The power relationships between the two are highly intricate and complex. This power is affected, for example, by the exclusive knowledge and expertise possessed by the nurse. In this, the patient is at a disadvantage. In some professions, this exclusivity of expertise is used to maintain power over those who have need of its service (e.g. medicine and law). Nursing's focus seems to lean more towards sharing expertise, thus empowering patients and 'turning the servant into the master' (Wilkes 1981).

This power relationship also affects the way nurses can act as advocates for patients. On the one hand, most nursing philosophies espouse this 'partnership' model in care, and urge nurses to act on patients' behalf when these patients are unable to do so themselves. It seems that this role for nurses is much more limited. Nurses also have obligations to employers and professional bodies. They have more power in the nurse–patient relationship – a power which can sometimes be used to suppress or control the patient's wishes (Sheehan 1994) or at least limit the nurse's objectivity. Therefore to see the named nurse as *the* patient's advocate is somewhat problematic. Rather, it seems more realistic to accept that there may occasionally be an appropriate advocacy role, but this is of limited scope in reality. Recognition of this limitation has led many settings to set up independent advocacy schemes, for example using voluntary organisations such as MIND or Age Concern.

The power relationship between nurse and patient is also subtly affected by the use of names. The giving of a name, for example, suggests that some degree of power is handed to the recipient from the donor (Gahagan 1984). Similarly, withholding the name implies a retention of a degree of power over the other. There has long been a debate in nursing over the appropriate use of names between nurses and patients (first name only? surnames only?) and yet there is remarkably little research into the subject. By implication, however, the revealing of the name in the named nurse concept, is significant. If the purpose of Patient's Charters is to empower patients by providing knowledge of available services, is there also an attempt to empower patients through the giving of nurses' names?

The notion of partnership assumes that both partners are willing, and able, to enter the relationship. The above discussion suggests that the power relationship between nurses and patients is far more complex than the rhetoric of the Patient's Charters implies.

The Patient's Charters indicate that the named nurse needs to be qualified. However, qualification is no guarantee that the nurse has all the skills and knowledge needed to deal with a patient's problems. Nurses need to be clear tht they are also competent to deal with any aspect of practice (UKCC 1992, 1993); if not they may have grounds for refusing to accept responsibility for a patient's care (RCN 1993).

Similarly, the degree to which patients may choose their nurse is highly problematic. Entering into a nurse–patient partnership implies that a degree of choice is available. In practice, the opportunities for patients to 'prefer' a particular nurse are extremely limited. The service tends to have limited capacity for flexible deployment of nurses. Also, the question of meeting a patient's choices becomes more difficult if, say, the patient refuses a nurse on the grounds of colour.

The Patient's Charters tend to convey an impression that there is considerable patient choice in care. In practice this may be very restricted and is certainly fraught with ethical and practical dilemmas when nurses or patients feel they have rights to choose or refuse to work with each other (RCN 1993; Wright 1993).

Conclusions

Within the confines of this chapter it has been possible to provide only an overview and discussion of some of the issues raised with the advent of the named nurse initiative. The reader who wishes to have more detailed information on organization and implementation is urged to obtain a copy of the Department of Health's guidance documents (Wright 1993).

Clearly the named nurse approach presents many challenges to nursing. Will nurses take the challenge, or will they, like Eveline in James Joyce's *The Dubliners* (Joyce 1904), retreat at the last moment, the allure of a new future being overwhelmed by fears of the unknown?

It presents a continued challenge to nurses to reappraise and explore the nurse–patient relationship. By exploring the nature of their alliance and partnership, there is tremendous potential for change – to the mutual benefit of both.

Named nursing is now being applied in all sectors of health care. The original charters were very hospital focused, but it is clear that there is now no branch of nursing where the named nurse is not being applied (DoH 1994; Wright 1993). There may be many motives for the initiative, but it is perhaps how nurses use it and exploit it to the benefit of patients and themselves that matters. For the first time in any country a government has made an explicit statement to its population about their entitlement to nursing. With all the reservations, complexities and uncertainties, some of which have been discussed in this chapter, it is clear that there is potential here for nurses not only to explore and expand their fundamental values in caring for another individual, but also their linchpin role in today's health services.

Reading guide

The government National Charter Standards on the named nurse concept may be found in the pamphlet *The Patient's Charter* (DoH 1992).

Further introductory reading material may be found in NHSE (1994), Hancock (1992), Cole and Davison (1992) and RCN (1992c). The defining document on the named nurse is perhaps Wright (1993).

The implementation of one approach to the named nurse concept, primary nursing, is discussed by Wright (1990) and Pearson (1988). A critical review of the literature on primary nursing and other ways of organizing nursing is provided by Ersser and Tutton (1991). A government document, *A Vision for the Future*, presents the named nurse concept in the context of a framework for the introduction of other nursing reforms (DoH NHSME 1993).

DoH NHSME (1993) *A Vision for the Future: The Nursing, Midwifery and Health Visiting Contribution to Health and Health Care.* HMSO, London.
Ersser, S. & Tutton, E. (1991) *Primary Nursing in Perspective.* Scutari Press, London.

References

Audit Commission (1991) *The Virtue of Patients.* Audit Commission, London.
Black, M. (1993) *The Growth of the Tameside Nursing Development Unit.* King's Fund Centre, London.
Briggs Report (1972) *Report of the Committee on Nursing.* Professor Asa Briggs (Chair). HMSO/DHSS, London.
Carr-Hill, R., Dixon, P., Gibbs, I., Griffiths, M., Higgins, M. McLaughan, D. & Wright K. *Skill Mix and the Effects on Nursing Care.* Centre for Health Economics, University of York.
Cole, A. & Davidson, I. (1992) Let's name names. *Nursing Times,* **88**(11), 24–7.
DoH (1992) *The Patient's Charter.* HMSO, London.
DoH (1994) *Testing the vision.* Department of Health, London.
Fanning, M. (1993) Naming Names. *Nursing Times,* **89**(44), 62–3.
Gahagan, J. (1984) *Social interaction and its management.* Methuen, London.
Hancock, C. (1992) The named nurse concept. *Nursing Standard* (special supplement) June.
Henderson, V. (1980) Preserving the essence of nursing. *Journal of Advanced Nursing,* **5**, 245–60.
Higgins, R. (1992) Consumerism and participation. *Senior Nurse,* **12**(5), 3–4.
Hugman, R. (1991) *Power in the Caring Professions.* Macmillan, London.
Hulme, K. (1986) *The Bone People.* Hodder & Stoughton, London.
Institute of Management Studies (1992) Nursing organisation in NHS and non-NHS hospitals. *Senior Nurse,* **12**(6), 30.
Joyce, J. (1904) Eveline. In: *The Dubliners* (reprinted 1992). Barnes and Noble, Dublin.
Kitson, A. (1988) On the concept of nursing care. In: *Ethical Issues in Caring.* (eds G. Fairbairn & S. Fairbairn). Avebury, Aldershot.
Menzies, I. (1961) The functioning of social systems as a defence against anxiety (reprinted 1988). In: *Containing Anxiety in Institutions.* (ed. I. Menzies-Lyth). Free Association Press, London.
NHSE (1994) *The Named Nurse, Midwife and Health Visitor – Checking that it happens.* National Health Service Executive, Leeds.
NIHPSO (1992) *A Charter for Patients and Clients.* Northern Ireland Health and Personal Social Services, Belfast.

Pearson, A. (ed.) (1988) *Primary Nursing.* Croom Helm, London.

Pearson, A. (1992) *Nursing at Burford, a Story of Change.* Scutari Press, London.

Pearson, A. & Vaughan, B. (1986) *Nursing Models for Nursing Practice.* Heinemann, London.

Pearson, A., Durand, I. & Punton, S. The feasibility and effectiveness of nursing beds. *Nursing Times* **84**(9), 48–50.

Peplau, H.E. (1952) *Interpersonal Relationships and Nursing.* Putnam, New York.

Robinson, K. (1992) Cited in Let's name names (Cole & Davidson). *Nursing Times*, **88**(11), 24–7.

RCN (1992a) *Approaches to Nursing Care.* Issues in Nursing and Health No. 13. Royal College of Nursing, London.

RCN (1992b) *The Value of Nursing.* Royal College of Nursing, London.

RCN (1992c) *The Named Nurse – Implications for Practice.* Issues in Nursing and Health No. 14. Royal College of Nursing, London.

RCN (1993) *Refusal to Nurse; Guidance for Nurses.* Issues in Nursing and Health No. 18. Royal College of Nursing, London.

Salvage, J. (1990) The theory and practice of the 'new nursing'. *Nursing Times*, **86**(4), 42–5.

Scottish Office (1991) *The Patient's Charter – a charter for health.* The Scottish Office, Edinburgh.

Sheehan, A. (1994) *A case study of patients, nurses and other professionals' perception of advocacy in the British and Dutch mental health systems.* MPhil Thesis, unpublished. University of Nottingham, Nottingham.

Snow, C. & Willard, P. (1989) *I'm Dying to Take Care of You.* Professional Counsellor Books, Redmond Washington.

UKCC (1992) *The Scope of Professional Practice.* United Kingdom Central Council for Nursing, Midwifery & Health Visiting, London.

UKCC (1993) *Code of Professional Conduct for the Nurse, Midwife and Health Visitor.* United Kingdom Central Council for Nursing, Midwifery and Health Visiting, London.

Welsh Office (1991) *Health – a Charter for Patients in Wales.* Welsh Office, Cardiff.

Wilkes, R. (1981) *Social Work with Under Valued Groups.* Tavistock, London.

Wright, S.G. (1989) *Changing Nursing Practice.* Edward Arnold, London.

Wright, S.G. (1990) *My Patient – My Nurse, the Practice of Primary Nursing.* Scutari Press, Harrow.

Wright, S.G. (ed.) (1993) *The Named Nurse, Midwife and Health Visitor.* NHSE, Leeds.

Commentary on Chapter 6

Terence Ryan

The named nurse is a utopian concept, highly desirable but not always achievable. In contemporary society it may be an expensive way of satisfying all patient demands. Health for all is another utopian endpoint to which the energies of all health professionals are directed. It is unlikely to happen as a result of natural evolution but requires professions concerned with health to learn about it and then to use their skills to achieve it. It too, however, is an expensive process and the main expense is for doctors as well as nurses. In many countries, nursing is the larger profession, but it is not so everywhere. It is probably true to say that the nurse is most often at the interface with the patient, whereas the doctor is frequently more distant. To achieve health for all there has to be involvement of central government, mostly the Department of Health, which receives advice from the medical profession more often than from the nursing profession. The individual at the periphery may more often receive advice from the nurse. The doctor usually has a longer training and is consequently more expensive to employ; the nurse is a cheaper option for delivery of health care in the periphery.

In this chapter Wright describes two ways of employing the nurse. One is to make them experts in a particular field and expect them to deliver that expertise to a large number of persons, hardly extending their skills beyond their sphere of expertise. The other, which is the named nurse, is in modern jargon more holistic, the patient's friend, educator and carer, delivering a range of expertise concerned with every aspect of the patient's illness and steering them towards good health.

Parallels can be drawn with the teaching profession. In the classroom there are teachers who are experts, but there have always been systems where the teacher stands and directs the entire class from the front, teaching only the subject of his or her expertise, while other systems have demanded small groups of pupils all doing their own thing at different rates, while the holistic teacher moves around directing events at each little table. Which system works best depends on the personality of the teacher as much as on their training. Not to be ignored is which system is most intellectually rewarding to which teacher. Every profession needs rewarding and some of the rewards should be intellectual.

In the medical profession we have generalists and specialists. In the UK the generalist is the highly respected General Practitioner, but in most parts of the world it is the specialist that the patient seeks for better management of their illness: 'I have been to see *my* dermatologist for *my* acne'. It is agreed that the overview of the GP is desirable, but it has to be supported by greater opportunities for professional growth and a wider range of skills. Some of these they can share, others they delegate. Sometimes when delegated to the nurse, they are perceived as a partnership!

When this chapter compares the named nurse with the nurse to whom a task is allocated, one inevitably asks who is the most expert 'generally' or in the 'specialist' field of the allocated task? One is told that both generalists and specialists can be 'named', just as one has one's own GP, and in hospital practice it is argued that the patient should be able to see the 'named' doctor of their choice.

Before coming to a conclusion about this chapter, I should explain my experience of task allocation versus the named nurse concept. In 1958, as a doctor in the Royal Army Medical Corps, we were faced with mass casualties, potentially from nuclear warfare. The health services were likely to be overwhelmed, and the only way to deal with this was procedure training. There were 20–30 essential procedures, and the soldier gradually learnt each of these. One soldier might be expert in applying splints, another capable of giving infusions, and that is as far as the expertise might go. It was thought to be the only way of dealing with mass casualties. In most parts of the world the health services are overwhelmed by masses of patients. That is one reason why the named nurse and health for all seem utopian.

In recent years I have been overseeing training schools for care of the skin and related diseases in Central America and in Africa. The nurse in Guatemala may be the only provider of health care for a population of around 15 000 people. She may have had only two years' training. There is no way in which she can be holistic. The nurses that I am training in Africa are even more thinly spread and we are providing a two-year training which makes them capable, in a country like Namibia, of creating programmes and advising governments. There is no way in which that nurse can be holistic at the interface with the patient.

Back home, where I head a dermatology department, we have created an environment in which the nurse can be expert, can be holistic, can be intellectually stimulated, while working at the interface with the patient. This is, however, an expensive programme in which nurses outnumber doctors, and on the ward they outnumber the patients. In this environment the named nurse provides not only patient satisfaction, but in the service in which a doctor is able to give only a few minutes of his or her time to each patient, the nurse is a substitute for the 'good physician' getting to know every aspect of the patient's background and instructing them how to cope with their illnesses.

If I was the Minister of Health, I would state that the named nurse is an ideal which, like health for all, we should aim for, but one cannot have it all the time and everywhere. In a health service which has to provide diagnosis of disease and is expected to provide high technology for often invasive procedures, there need to be doctors capable of overseeing such procedures, often with a long and specialised training, which is rewarded by a high salary. The management of disease after the diagnosis has been made and after invasive procedures have taken place, requires a named nurse at the interface with the patient. How many of these we can afford depends on keeping the salaries down. The named nurse will expect professional growth to acquire a wider range of skill and consequently she or he will expect a salary higher than that, and will deserve it. Some jobs are still best delegated to those who have learnt one or two procedures only, and this can be a more cost-effective way of providing the health service.

Emphasizing that cost has to be taken into account is a very contemporary way of looking at the problem. In order to provide job satisfaction, one has to seek beyond the provision of salary to other kinds of rewards which are derived from good working relationships between the professions, good working environments, and intellectual attainment. In this context, if the named nurse is to be optimally achieved, the concept should be examined, not merely in the framework of the nursing profession, but in the framework of partnerships with the medical profession and others, and rewards which are not merely financial and working environments which are not merely a bedside, must be taken into account. For the patient or pupil to have their own doctor, nurse or tutor at all times is an expensive option, and task allocation or expertise in a procedure is a cost- effective alternative when faced by overwhelming demands. A profession which states that all traffic lights should be replaced by roundabouts, would have to return to traffic lights when the traffic exceeds the capacity of the roundabout. This should not mean that all roundabouts become obsolete everywhere. The nursing profession must see the benefits of both task allocation and the named-nurse where appropriate to demands and resources.

7 ◆ Patient Controlled Analgesia and the Concept of Patient-Centred Care

Veronica J. Thomas

Over the past three decades, the patient's role has changed from being predominantly passive to being dynamic. Nurses' roles have also changed from a focus on caring for dependent patients to that of partnerships with the patients in the provision of care. The Nursing Process (Henderson 1961; Roper *et al.* 1990) was perhaps the first nursing model that favoured an individualized, patient-centred approach to care. The philosophy inherent in this type of care considers patients to be autonomous and central to the decision making which affects their health and wellbeing (Jewell 1994). Patient controlled analgesia (PCA), a technique which allows the patients to control their own level of pain by self-administering small bolus doses of opioids intravenously, personifies this approach to patient care. In allowing individualized therapy and facilitating personal control, PCA is seen as an important innovation.

This chapter will discuss the management of acute postoperative pain and the ways in which it has been revolutionized by PCA. I will also consider the extent to which this analgesic method embodies the philosophy of patient-centred care.

Inadequate postoperative pain management

When a patient is extremely ill and dependent, it is easy for the health care professional to 'take over'. The problem with this approach is that it easily becomes extended beyond the point of necessity to a situation where both the carer and the patient find it difficult to relinquish the dominant and dependent roles (Benner & Wrubel 1988). This is a situation that has existed (and to some extent still exists) within the context of post-operative pain control for the past 25 years. Pain after surgery continues to evade reliable clinical management (Cohen 1980; Khun *et al.* 1990; Royal College of Surgeons & College of Anaesthetists 1990; Seers 1987; Weis *et al.* 1983) and remains the most common complaint following surgical operations. Apart from the misery and suffering, postoperative pain is likely to bring a succession of avoidable complications that may impede the patient's recovery.

Inadequate treatment of postoperative pain is caused by many factors but the attitude of patients and health care professionals is seen as a great hindrance. Although pain is considered a subjective experience, validation is sought from physiological signs (objectively), and often the patient is not consulted. When such physiological signs are not apparent, the patient's report of pain is sometimes met with, 'nonsense, it couldn't possibly hurt' or 'it isn't time yet'. These words reveal the misconception that doctors and nurses believe that they, rather than the patient, are the authority on the patient's pain.

McCaffery (1979) believes that patients have various pain rights which include:

(1) to decide the duration and intensity of pain they wish to tolerate;
(2) to be informed of all possible methods of pain relief available;
(3) the choice of which methods they wish to use.

This self-determination is one of the values which underlies patient-centred care and is inherent in the ethical code which nurses profess (Copp 1985). As stated earlier, patient-centred care places the patient at the heart of the health care decisions. Pain, as a highly complex and subjective symptom, truly warrants this conviction; however, the bulk of the evidence suggests that patients' self-determination is not generally sought in the management of postoperative pain.

The conventional method of administering pain relief

Because of low cost and ease of administration, the majority of post-operative patients are treated with intermittent intramuscular injection (IMI) or subcutaneous injections of a fixed dose of opioid. Many researchers (Austin *et al.* 1980; Royal College of Surgeons and College of Anaesthetists Working Party Report 1990) have repeatedly pointed to the inadequacies inherent in these conventional analgesic regimes.

Fig. 7.1 demonstrates the usual cycle experienced by a patient requesting pain relief. Many factors contribute to substantial delays between the time pain is perceived and when relief is obtained. The patient in pain initiates the cycle by calling the nurse. Unfortunately the work demands of the clinical setting, time and staff shortages all contribute to the delay between the patient report of pain and its relief. The delay in responding has been estimated to be at least 30 minutes (Vache 1982). Yet the majority of patients are not aware of this delay. In a recent study, Owen *et al.* (1990) demonstrated that 75% of surgical patients expected that when they requested analgesia, they would receive it immediately. The lag between demand and response is a failing of this conventional method which significantly contributes to poor pain management and undermines the logic of patient-centred care.

In many hospitals the standard prescription order says PRN (*pro re nata*, or 'as needed'), in an attempt to have the right dose delivered when most needed. However, such orders are often subject to a minimum interval between doses, which are decided in advance by the prescriber. This is clearly not patient-centred since it is generally not individualized according to need. Melzack (1990) argues that this form of prescribing often results in confrontation between the patient and

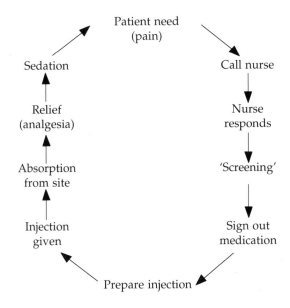

Fig. 7.1 The cyclic character of conventional analgesic therapy (Graves *et al.* 1983. Reproduced from *Annals of Internal Medicine*).

the nurse. The nurse expects the analgesia to last for four to six hours and the patient, whose pain has returned earlier than expected, is in agony and pleads to have another injection.

Health care professionals, particularly nurses, have prime responsibility for providing effective pain relief for surgical patients. However, from the above discussion it is evident that there are a host of staff, patient and organizational variables interacting to hinder a patient-centred approach to pain management.

Patient controlled analgesia (PCA)

A well accepted definition of pain proposed for use by nurses in clinical practice, and which strongly supports the philosophy of patient-centred care, is offered by McCaffery (1979). She states that pain is 'what the experiencing person says it is, existing when the experiencing person says it does'. If we accept this definition of pain, then it naturally follows that we should entrust the patient with the means of relieving it. In addressing the problem of inadequately controlled postoperative pain, researchers have moved away from the search for the perfect analgesic, and moved towards the development of more effective routes of administration. To this end they have centred on the necessity to integrate the knowledge of the pharmacokinetics of the analgesic agents with the response of the individual patient to that agent, as well as the personal experience of the patient.

PCA is a method of pain control in which these factors are fully recognized (Thomas & Rose 1993). It is a most exciting development which hands over the control of pain to the patient and bypasses the delays and deficiencies of the conventional pain relief method. The PCA system originally developed out of an attempt to measure pain accurately and objectively. In 1968, Sechzer considered on-demand analgesia to be an excellent way to measure pain because of the observed positive correlation between the degree of pain reported and the amount of analgesic requested. Forrest *et al.* (1970) developed this idea further by suggesting that the patient's demand for analgesia should be incorporated into a method for the control of postoperative pain.

The PCA system consists of a syringe pump and a timing device. The patient activates the system by pressing a button, causing a small dose of analgesic to be delivered into the venous system. Simultaneously a lockout device is activated ensuring that another dose cannot be delivered until the first dose has had time to exert its full effect. Recent development of PCA technology appears to have followed two main streams. One is the development of increasingly sophisticated bedside drug delivery systems and the other is production of smaller devices suitable for ambulatory use.

Although PCA has been used extensively in the USA, its use in the UK has been rather more limited until very recently (Thomas & Rose 1993). However, its efficacy in controlling postoperative pain and its popularity among patients and staff (Thomas 1993), should ensure that its appropriate usage becomes more widespread.

PCA as an efficient means of controlling postoperative pain

Numerous research reports indicate that PCA is a great improvement on the conventional PRN intramuscular method (for example, Delbos *et al.* 1993; Kerri-Szanto & Heaman 1972; Notcutt & Morgan 1990; O'Connor *et al.* 1993; Slattery *et al.* 1983; Thomas *et al.* 1990; Thomas *et al.* 1993). PCA is currently the ultimate patient-centred pain management technique because it allows patients to determine when and how much analgesic they receive, and secondly it allows determination of a minimum blood drug concentration associated with effective analgesic concentration and minimum side effects (MEAC) despite great interpatient variability (Ferrante 1990).

In the earliest comparative study, Kerri-Szanto and Heaman (1972) found that 40% of patients receiving intramuscular therapy complained of pain in the 48 hours after surgery compared to 5% of those receiving pain control via PCA. More recent research has produced similar results. For example, Thomas *et al.* (1993) found significant differences in the efficacy of PCA and IMI with superior pain control being associated with PCA for the first 24 hours after surgery. Similarly, O'Connor *et al.* (1993) found that within the first four hours after surgery, patients receiving IM injections experienced 80% of the worst pain they could imagine, as compared to 30% among the PCA groups.

A few researchers (Smith 1984; Thomas *et al.* 1990, 1993; Thomas

1991) have also found that PCA provides pain relief with a lower total dose of analgesic agent. In these studies patients receiving adequate control via intramuscular therapy were given in the region of 30% more opioids than that required by patients controlling their own analgesia. In contrast Slattery *et al.* (1983) found that patients receiving the traditional PRN treatment following abdominal surgery received much less analgesia than the PCA group. However, they also reported more pain, which provides evidence to support the claim that the PRN method is not as flexible as was originally intended because it is sometimes interpreted to mean as little as possible (Mather 1983).

PCA can also be claimed to be superior to the more conventional postoperative analgesic regimes in bringing about a reduction in hospital stay. A number of studies (Clark *et al.* 1989; Thomas *et al.* 1990, 1993; Thomas 1991) have shown that PCA patients are discharged on average two days earlier than IMI patients. This suggests that PCA promotes recovery; an explanation for this is that PCA provides an increased sense of control, which promotes a sense of wellbeing (Thomas & Rose 1993).

The overall impression gained from the literature on post-operative and other types of acute pain (see Thomas & Rose 1993 for a full review) is that PCA is superior to the conventional IMI method. This superiority may, in part, be attributable to PCA's ability to provide a constant level of pain relief. As we have already noted, it is also likely to be partly due to psychological factors such as being 'in control'. There are, however, individuals who do not want to exercise control (Miller 1979; Thomas 1991; Wallston *et al.* 1978; Wilson & Bennett 1984). Although in general these reluctant participants constitute the minority, it is important to a patient-centred philosophy that their styles of coping are taken into consideration.

PCA enhances personal control

The importance of control in our lives is seldom considered until it is taken away (Egan 1990) and control over events is important for both the safety and comfort of the individual. There is also evidence that lack of control (Peck 1986) is intrinsically aversive and anxiety provoking. Most individuals view impending surgery as a stressor involving loss of immediate control, pain, and the potential loss of ability to resume normal activities (Auerbach 1979). In the surgical situation there are limits to the amount of control that patients can exercise over aversive events since these events are regulated by nursing and medical staff.

In attempting to reduce the level of pre and postoperative stress, researchers have tried to enhance patients' sense of control through the use of information (Hayward 1975; Owens & Hutlemeyer 1982), cognitive strategies (Langer *et al.* 1975; Ridgeway & Mathews 1982; Wells *et al.* 1986) and behavioural control interventions (Thomas 1991; Wilson 1981); for example, information given to patients before an operation allows them to interpret and understand their surroundings and circumstances, and this helps them to anticipate the events which occur during the postoperative period.

The ability to understand and to anticipate engenders a feeling of control and reduces helplessness (Lazarus 1966). Since helplessness is a major component of anxiety (Mandler 1972), anxiety is reduced. Pain after an operation is beyond the influence of the subject and this lack of control is a major source of suffering in itself. Giving patients a PCA device that allows them to modulate pain levels is a humane step towards returning to them some modicum of control over their lives (Egan 1990), and is perhaps the ultimate in patient-centred approach.

Thompson (1981) defined control as the belief that one has at one's disposal a response that can influence the aversiveness of an event. This definition is very useful because it recognizes that control does not have to be exercised (potential control) for it to be effective, and that it does not even have to be real, just perceived, for it to have effects. However, an important question is, why is it that this belief in personal control is so effective in reducing postoperative pain? Several theorists (Johnson *et al.* 1971; Miller 1979; Seligman & Maier 1967) have proposed that control strategies reduce pain and anxiety because they allow the person to predict some important aspects of the situation, such as when the painful experience will occur, when it will end and what it will feel like. All these theorists have made the implicit assumption that the person has a pivotal role to play in managing their pain and stress.

Thompson (1981) states that a common theme uniting all the literature on control is the meaning of the event for the individual. It has long been noted in the study of pain that the meaning of an injury or its consequences dramatically affect the amount of pain felt (Beecher 1956). On the other hand, Arntz and Schmidt (1989) suggest that it is the inferred harmfulness of the pain which is the central issue. Control over pain causes changes in the meaning and hence the way it is experienced. They further propose that pain that can be controlled is perceived as harmless and therefore has a different significance for the patient. Pain that cannot be controlled is considered to be harmful and the individual perceives himself to be helpless since nothing can be done about it.

Miller's (1979) minimax hypothesis states that patients with controlling responses (whether they are actual or perceived) believe that postoperative pain will not become so bad that they are unable to cope. The reason for this is that they have at their disposal the means to bring about relief. This theory captures one important dimension of meaning: the assurance that pain will not be beyond the limits of one's endurance. This endurable–unendurable aspect of meaning could be seen as analogous to Arntz and Schmidt's (1989) harmless–harmful dichotomy in the perception of pain, and could perhaps help to explain many of the effects of informational, cognitive and behavioural control interventions in the postoperative patient. It is particularly useful in explaining the findings that show that PCA patients use less analgesic medication and yet report less pain.

PCA gives patients both a behavioural control and a decisional control, since the patient engages in an active behaviour which modifies the pain level, and he/she can decide whether or not to press the button. It appears that a device like PCA brings another important aspect to the endurable–unendurable dimension: the right to decide what is and what is not endurable. The fact that some individuals use less analgesia suggests that this knowledge of self control increases one's ability to endure more.

In summary, it seems that perceived control minimizes the post-operative pain experience and anxiety. Actual controlling responses such as are afforded by PCA have dramatic effects in speeding recovery as well. However, in a culture where it is seen as essential for patients to be actively involved in the decision making process (Biley 1992), we are in danger of losing the patient-centred philosophy by putting control into the hands of reluctant participants. It is important to recognize that some individuals do not want to be autonomous or actively involved, and a blanket approach to PCA allocation could be a retrograde step.

My experiences in the clinical use of PCA

Although PCA allows the patient to take control, it is my firm belief (borne out by practical experience) that nursing expertise is crucial for its successful implementation. Nurses can provide explanations and practical demonstration which will enable patients to use this method efficiently. Proper monitoring of patients by nurses is essential. Regular monitoring of patients' respiratory rate is important because of the potential risk of respiratory depression. Another important reason for monitoring the patient is to determine whether pain is being controlled. It should not be assumed that good pain control is being achieved simply because a PCA system is attached to the patient.

Some patients may not use PCA because they are worried about addiction or because they have traditional attitudes concerning pain relief and, as a consequence, believe that the nurse should control analgesia. Thus unless individual assessments of patients using PCA are made, PCA may become a victim of the same inadequacies as the conventional intramuscular method. Therefore in assisting the introduction of PCA in a district hospital, I have recommended that the nurses assess the patient's level of pain at regular intervals as well as providing information to allay fears and reassure patients about overdose and addiction.

During the initial stages of PCA's more extensive introduction in the hospital, many nurses were concerned about dealing with new machinery and about the possibility of patients being overmedicated or becoming addicted. Education programmes concerning the function and use of PCA quickly dispelled these concerns. There were, however, a few nurses who remained reluctant to relinquish control to their patients. This attitude was obvious when some nurses were observed pushing the button for their patients! This problem disappeared when it was explained that NCA (nurse controlled analgesia) defeats the objective of PCA. As nurses and doctors became used to PCA, they quickly recognized its advantages and accepted it unreservedly. A survey of nurses' and doctors' views towards PCA points to this acceptance, demonstrating that the majority liked the autonomy and comfort it gave their patients (Thomas 1993).

PCA has also been found to be associated with a time saving of 42 minutes per patient per day of nurses' time. This has contributed tremendously to nurses' acceptance of this analgesic method. In a busy surgical ward this represents a significant amount of time. The primary message I have tried to convey to the nursing staff is that, this time, gain could be used to improve communication between nurses, patients and their relatives. In so doing I have tried to emphasize that nurse–patient contact is of paramount importance to patients and this should not be forgotten with PCA.

Although patients are generally satisfied with the effectiveness of relief obtained from PCA, effective analgesia may not necessarily be related to patient satisfaction. Some patients may prefer more nursing attention (Koh & Thomas 1994), whilst fear of overdose may result in underuse of PCA and the patient experiencing more pain than with IM injections (Dodson 1985). The extent to which patients accept and use PCA is dependent on their attitudes and beliefs about pain and its relief, in other words their psychology.

Psychological components of PCA

Whilst in general terms PCA does appear to be superior to IMI, this cannot be taken to mean that PCA functions optimally for all patients. In a recent study Murphy *et al.* (1993) found that a small proportion of surgical patients were unwilling to use PCA despite encouragement. Although personality variables were not measured it is highly likely that this reluctance was influenced by psychological factors. When individual differences in the preferences for control are taken into consideration the patient-centred philosophy will be apparent and the effect of control in reducing pain becomes significantly enhanced.

It is well recognized that psychological factors play a significant role in the perception and tolerance of pain as well as in the willingness to communicate the discomfort and distress caused by pain (Johnston 1980; Melzack & Wall 1988; Sternbach 1978), yet few researchers have acknowledged their important implications in relation to PCA. This seems extraordinary when one considers that PCA requires full patient co-operation and participation (Thomas & Rose 1993). The research which addresses psychological issues concerning PCA is limited to three studies. These have examined the effect of patient's locus of control, coping styles and level of anxiety.

The tendency to seek opportunities for personal control in a situation is a personality disposition that varies from person to person and is called locus of control (Rotter 1975). The multi-dimensional health locus of control (MHLC) (Wallston *et al.* 1978) inventory defines three areas of control: internality, powerful others, and chance externality.

'Internals' believe that their own health is under their control and is a result of their behaviour, while 'externals' believe that luck, fate, chance, or 'powerful others' have control over health. With respect to PCA, Johnson *et al.* (1988) measured locus of health control (with the MHLC) and found that surgical patients with an external locus of control experienced higher pain scores and a greater degree of dissatisfaction with PCA. On the other hand, patients who believed that their health is under their own control (internal locus of control) experienced lower levels of pain and a greater satisfaction with PCA.

Coping style refers to characteristic ways of dealing with stressful situations, which different individuals adopt. Generally people either seek further information about the threat ('monitors' or 'sensitizers') or they distract themselves from threat-relevant information ('Blunters' or 'Avoiders'). Monitors are thought to have a high need for control and to utilise information as a means of gaining some degree of control (Miller 1979; Miller *et al.* 1989). Blunters, in contrast, have a low desire for control and cope better by psychologically absenting themselves from threatening information. According to this theory patients who adopt an avoidant/blunting strategy would be unlikely to agree to use PCA and may become distressed postoperatively if required to do so. On the other hand, patients who are monitors are likely to benefit from the additional control which PCA provides.

In a recent study Thomas (1991) attempted to identify categories of surgical patients who benefit maximally from PCA, by measuring preoperative anxiety and coping style using Miller's behavioural style scale (Miller 1987). This revealed a negative correlation between coping style score and pain experience among patients using PCA and is consistent with findings by Wilson and Bennett (1984). Therefore patients with low monitoring style scores, which reflects a low desire for control, did not exercise the control they were given with PCA and as a consequence experienced a significant amount of pain. In addition, patients who were highly anxious before surgery achieved greater benefits (in terms of pain reduction) than patients with low levels of anxiety.

In summary, if a patient does not normally acknowledge a degree of personal control and responsibility for his/her own health, allocation to a PCA regime may be a source of stress to the patient and prove less beneficial than more conventional methods.

Criteria for the allocation of PCA

These psychological studies suggest that for all its advantages PCA does not work in a simple and consistent manner for everyone. Psychological factors relevant to the experience of postoperative pain, such as anxiety, neuroticism, locus of control and coping style, are clearly important. The problem is how to identify the psychological profile of a patient who will use PCA effectively in order to achieve its maximum benefits. It is important to do this not only to maximize pain relief for patients but also to ensure efficient allocation of a scarce resource. PCA equipment is costly and as a consequence constraints are placed on its availability. Therefore it is very important that the available PCA systems are used as efficiently as possible. In a climate of scarcity, attention should be focused on the method of allocation of PCA systems. I am engaged in research to address this problem.

Conclusions

Establishing the patient as central to the decision making process has been an important and welcome change in the philosophy of nursing care generally, and in the management of postoperative pain in particular. PCA can reduce pain, promote tolerance and facilitate speedy recovery. As such it can be seen to have brought about a small revolution in postoperative pain management and will continue to do so if proper assessment of individual preferences is undertaken. Placing a control device (in the form of PCA) into everyone's hand without questioning whether it is appropriate is not employing an individualized approach to care. In this way PCA could become a victim of the same inadequacies as conventional methods, i.e. the nurse or the doctor are the authority on patients' pain control.

Irrespective of the method used to provide pain relief, postoperative patients require more than the mere provision of analgesic medication. They require to be treated as individuals. PCA's ability to truly embody patient-centred philosophy can only be realised when health care professionals recognize that if they are to take seriously patients' rights to participate they must show greater respect for individuality when allocating these analgesic systems. I am continuing work in an attempt to develop a quick and easy questionnaire method which can be used as a basis for deciding which patient will achieve maximal benefit from PCA.

References

Arntz, A. & Schmidt, A.J.M. (1989) Perceived control and the experience of pain. In: *Stress, Personal Control and Health* (eds A. Steptoe & A. Appels). Wiley, Chichester.

Auerbach, S.M. (1979) Pre-operative preparation for surgery. A review of recent research and future prospects. In: *Research in Psychology and Medicine*, vol. 2, social aspects: attitudes, communication, care & training (eds D.J. Osborne, M.M. Gruneberg & J.R. Eiser), pp. 345–9. Academic Press, New York.

Austin, K.L., Stapleton, J.V. & Mather, L.E. (1980) Multiple intramuscular injections: a major source of variability in analgesic response to meperidine. *Pain*, **8**, 47–62.

Beecher, H.K. (1956) Relationship of significance of wound to pain experienced. *Journal of the American Medical Association*, **161**, 1609–13.

Benner, P. & Wrubel, J. (1988) *The Primacy of Caring: Stress and Coping in Health and Illness*. Addison-Wesley, California.

Biley, F.C. (1992) Some determinants that effect patient participation in decision making about nursing care. *Journal of Advanced Nursing*, **17**, 414–21.

Clark, E., Hodsman, N. & Kenny, G. (1989) Improved postoperative recovery with patient controlled analgesia. *Nursing Times*, **85**(9), 54–5.

Cohen, F.L. (1980) Postsurgical pain relief: patient's status and nurses' medication choices. *Pain*, **9**, 265–74.

Copp, L.A. (1985) Pain, ethics and the negotiation of values. In: Perspectives on Pain (ed. L.A. Copp) *Recent Advances in Nursing Series*, **11**, 137–49.

Delbos, M., Chandeclerc, M., Chaubard C., *et al.* (1993) *Twenty five months of PCA in a French Private Hospital*. Book of Abstracts, 7th World Congress on Pain, 22–27 August, p. 392. IASP Publications, Seattle.

Dodson, M.E. (1985) *The Management of Postoperative Pain*. Current Topics in Anaesthesia Series, vol. 8. Edward Arnold, London.

Egan, K.J. (1990) What does it mean to be a patient in control? In: *Patient Controlled Analgesia* (eds F.M. Ferrante, G.W. Ostheimer & G. Covino), pp. 17–26. Blackwell Science, Boston.

Ferrante, F.M. (1990) Patient Controlled Analgesia as a Research Tool. In: *Patient Controlled Analgesia* (eds F.M. Ferrante, G.W. Ostheimer & G. Covino), pp. 61–9. Blackwell Science, Boston.

Forrest, W.H., Smethurst, P.W.R. & Kienitz, M.B. (1970) Self-administration of intravenous analgesics. *Anaesthesiology*, **33**, 363–5.

Graves, D.A., Foster, T.S., Batenhorst, R.L., Bennett, R.L. & Baumann, T.J. (1983) Patient controlled analgesia. *Annals of Internal Medicine*, **99**, 360–66.

Hayward, J. (1975) *Information: a prescription against pain*. The Study of Nursing Care Reports, series 2, No. 5. Royal College of Nursing, London.

Henderson, V. (1966) *The Nature of Nursing – A Definition and its Implications for Practice, Research and Education*. Macmillan, New York.

Jewell, S.E. (1994) Patient participation: what does it mean to nurses? *Journal of Advanced Nursing*, **19**, 433–8.

Johnson, J.E., Leventhal, H. & Dabbs, J.M. (1971) Contribution of emotional and instrumental response processes in adaptation to surgery. *Journal of Personality and Social Psychology*, **20**, 55–64.

Johnson, J.E., Rice, V.H., Fuller, S.S. & Endress, M.P. (1978) Sensory information, instruction in coping strategy and recovery from surgery. *Research in Nursing and Health*, **1**, 4–7.

Johnson, L.R., Ferrante, F.M., Magnani, B.J. & Rocco, A.G. (1988) Psychological modifiers of PCA efficacy. *Pain*, **39**, 17–22.

Johnston, M. (1980) Anxiety in surgical patients. *Psychological Medicine*, **10**, 145–52.

Keeri-Szanto, M. & Heaman, S. (1972) Postoperative demand analgesia. *Surgery Gynaecology & Obstetrics*, **134**, 647–51.

Khun, S., Cooke, K., Collins, M., *et al.* (1990) Perceptions of pain relief after surgery. *British Medical Journal*, **300**, 1687–90.

Koh, P. & Thomas, V.J. (1994) Patient controlled analgesia: does time saved by PCA improve patient satisfaction with nursing care? *Journal of Advanced Nursing*, **20**, 61–70.

Langer, R.S., Janis, I. & Wolfer, J. (1975) Reduction of psychological stress in surgical patients. *Journal of Experimental and Social Psychology*, **11**, 155–65.

Lazarus, R.S. (1966) *Psychological Stress and Coping Process*. McGraw-Hill, New York.

Mandler, G. (1972) Helplessness: theory and research in anxiety. In: *Anxiety: Current Trends in Theory and Research* (ed. C.D. Spielberger). Academic Press, New York.

Mather, L.E. (1983) Pharmacokinetic and pharmacodynamic factors influencing the choice, dose and route of opiates for acute pain. *Clinics in Anaesthesiology*, **1**(1), 17–40.

McCaffery, M. (1979) *Nursing Management of the Patient in Pain.* J.B. Lipincott, Philadelphia.

Melzack, R. (1990) The tragedy of needless pain. *Scientific American*, February, 27–33.

Melzack, R. & Wall, P.D. (1988) *The Challenge of Pain*, pp. 15–33. Penguin, Harmondsworth.

Miller, S.M. (1979) Controllability and human stress: method, evidence and theory. *Behaviour, Research and Theory*, **17**, 287–304.

Miller, S.M. (1987) Monitoring and blunting: validation of a questionnaire to assess different styles of coping with stress. *Journal of Personality and Social Psychology*, **52**, 345–53.

Miller, S.M., Coombs, C. & Stoddard, E. (1989) Information, coping and control in patients undergoing surgery and stressful procedures. In: *Stress, Personal Control and Health* (eds A. Steptoe & A. Appels), pp. 107–29). Wiley, Chichester.

Mischel, W. (1979) On the interface of cognition and personality. *American Psychologist*, **34**, 740.

Murphy, D.F., Grazioti, P., Chalkiadias, G. *et al.* (1993) *Patient controlled analgesia for postoperative pain relief: a comparison with nurse controlled intravenous opioids.* Book of Abstracts, 7th World Congress on Pain, 22–27 August, p. 393. IASP Publications, Seattle.

Notcutt, W.G. & Morgan, R.J.M. (1990) Introducing patient-controlled analgesia for postoperative pain control into a district general hospital. *Anaesthesia*, **45**, 401–6.

O'Connor, M., Warwick, P. & Culpeper, V.E. (1993) *Evaluation of the effectiveness of an acute pain team.* Book of Abstracts, 7th World Congress on Pain, 22–27 August, p. 394. IASP Publications, Seattle.

Owen, H., McMillan, V. & Rogowski, D. (1990) Postoperative pain therapy: a survey of patients' expectations and their experiences. *Pain*, **41**, 303–7.

Owens, J.F. & Hutlemeyer, C.M. (1982) The effect of preoperative intervention of delirium on cardiac surgical patients. *Nursing Research*, **31**, 60–62.

Peck, C.L. (1986) Psychological factors in acute pain management. In: *Acute Pain Management* (eds M.J. Cousins & G.D. Phillips), pp. 251–74. Churchill Livingstone, Edinburgh.

Ridgeway, V. & Mathews, A. (1982) Psychological preparation for surgery: a comparison of methods. *British Journal of Clinical Psychology*, **21**, 271–80.

Roper, N., Logan, W.W. & Tierney, A.J. (1990) *The Model of Nursing Based on a Model of Living* (3rd ed). Churchill Livingstone, Edinburgh.

Rotter, J.B. (1975) Some problems and misconceptions related to the locus of control. *Journal of Consulting and Clinical Psychology*, **43**, 56–67.

Royal College of Surgeons and College of Anaesthetists (1990) Commission of the Provisions of Surgical Services. Report of the Working Party on Pain After Surgery.

Sechzer, P.H. (1968) Objective measurement of pain. *Anaesthesiology*, **29**, 209–10.

Seers, C.J. (1987) *Pain, anxiety and recovery in patients undergoing surgery.* Unpublished PhD thesis, Kings College, University of London.

Seligman, M.E.P. & Maier, S.F. (1967) Failure to escape traumatic shock. *Journal of Experimental Psychology*, **74**, 1–9.

Slattery, P.J., Harmer, M. & Rosen, M. (1983) An open comparison between routine and self-administered postoperative pain relief. *Annals of the Royal College of Surgeons*, **65**, 13–19.

Smith, G. (1984) Cardiff palliator. *British Journal of Anaesthesia*, **56**, 311.

Sternbach, R.A. (ed.) (1978) *The Psychology of Pain.* Raven Press, New York.

Thomas, V.J. (1991) *Personality characteristics of patients and the effectiveness of patient controlled analgesia.* Unpublished PhD thesis, Goldsmiths' College, University of London.

Thomas, V.J. (1993) The views of patients and staff concerning patient controlled analgesia. *Nursing Standard*, **7**(28), 37–9.

Thomas, V.J. & Rose, F.D. (1993) Patient controlled analgesia: a new method for old. *Journal of Advanced Nursing*, **18**, 1719–26.

Thomas, V.J., Heath, M.L. & Rose, F.D. (1990) Effect of psychological variables and pain relief system on postoperative pain experience. *British Journal of Anaesthesia*, **64**, 388–9.

Thomas, V.J., Rose, F.D., Heath, M.L. & Flory, P. (1993) A multidimensional comparison of nurse and patient controlled analgesia in the management of acute post surgical pain. *Medical Science Research*, **21**, 379–81.

Thompson, S.C. (1981) Will it hurt less if I can control it? A complex answer to a simple question. *Psychological Bulletin*, **90**, 89–101.

Utting, J.E. & Smith, J.M. (1979) Postoperative analgesia. *Anaesthesia*, **34**, 320–32.

Vache, E. (1982) Inadequate treatment of pain in hospitalised patients. *New England Journal of Medicine*, **307**, 55.

Wallston, K.A., Wallston, B.S. & Devillis, R. (1978) Development of multi-dimensional health locus of control scales. *Health Education Monograph*, **6**, 160–70.

Weis, O.F., Sriwatanakul, K. & Alloza, J.L. *et al.* (1983) Attitudes of patients, house staff, and nurses toward postoperative analgesic care. *Anaesthesia and Analgesia*, **62**(1), 70–74.

Wells, J.K., Howard, G.S., Nowlin, W.F. & Vargas, M.J. (1986) Pre-surgical anxiety and post-surgical pain and adjustment: effects of stress inoculation procedure. *Journal of Consulting and Clinical Psychology*, **54**, 831–5.

Wilson, J.F. (1981) Behavioural preparation for surgery: benefit or harm? *Journal of Behavioural Medicine*, **4**, 79–102.

Wilson, J.F. & Bennett, R.L. (1984) Coping styles, medication use and pain scores in patients using PCA for postoperative pain. *Abstract Anaesthesiology*, **61**, A193.

Commentary on Chapter 7

David Rose

Patient Controlled Analgesia (PCA) works! That much is clear from Thomas' very clear account of the literature. Of course she notes the important caveats – of which more later – and PCA is certainly not a complete answer to the problems of pain control. However, for most patients PCA represents a measurable improvement on traditional methods of dealing with postoperative pain. PCA has been shown to be associated with lower pain ratings, reduce analgesic consumption, shorter hospitalization and greater patient satisfaction. It is a powerful weapon in the armoury of those concerned with the control of pain. Yet, as Thomas observes, in this country its use has been relatively limited. Why has it taken so long for PCA to be accepted, and why, even now, is it not much more widely used? In this commentary on Thomas' chapter I should like to explore this question further.

A somewhat prosaic explanation might lie in financial considerations. Thomas notes that PCA equipment is costly – certainly in comparison with the costs of syringes and hypodermics needed for intramuscular and subcutaneous injections. Set against the higher initial outlay, however, must be the cost savings identified by Thomas. The reductions in nurses' time (in the region of 40 minutes per patient per day) and in length of hospitalization (PCA patients are discharged on average two days earlier than patients given the traditional intramuscular treatment), represent a considerable financial saving when looked at across the whole population of patients undergoing surgery in a single hospital in one year. A rough calculation would suggest that PCA machines would soon pay for themselves and, thereafter, represent a saving. Financial constraints would seem to be an insufficient explanation.

A more likely explanation lies in a degree of confusion about the technique's rationale. There are both general and specific arguments for PCA. The former are concerned with a patient-centred approach to pain treatment and the latter with giving the patient control over that treatment. Understandably it is the latter which Thomas emphasizes in her chapter. However, both types of arguments are important if we are to understand why a pain control method with such intuitive appeal has not been greeted with quite as much enthusiasm as we might have expected.

The rationale for a patient-centred approach to the control of pain is clear and derives from developments in our understanding of pain itself, which have undergone a revolution in the last 50 years. Up until the 1960s the model of pain taught in the medical curriculum derived from the 'specificity' theory which, itself, had changed little since it was first proposed by Descartes in the 1600s. Essentially pain was thought to be subserved by a simple and automatic sensory system. Noxious stimulation fed in at the periphery would activate pain centres in the brain which then produced the experience of pain. The alternative names for the theory, push button or alarm bell theory, described it well.

Given this sort of model of pain the approach to pain control was straightforward, at least in principle. The aim of all pain control interventions was to reduce the level of ascending activity in the pain pathway. However this was attempted, the treatment was something which was done to the patient's pain pathway. Whilst some patients might be more stoical than others in their acceptance of pain, there was no reason to suppose that to involve them in their own treatment would alter their level of pain in any way.

Of course clinicians knew that the treatments which followed logically from this specificity model were often of limited value in practice. In response the model was developed giving rise to various 'pattern' theories. However, the emphasis was on reformulation of the proposed peripheral input mechanisms, rather than on elaboration of the importance of the patient's own experience.

The revolution came in the 1960s with the gate control theory of pain (Melzack & Wall 1965). Melzack and Wall concentrated on pain experience which did not comply with the specificity theory's predicted correlation between the strength of the noxious stimulation and the intensity of the pain experience. They acknowledged that in clinical situations there was often no obvious correlation at all. One of the ways in which they sought to explain this was to emphasize the role of the patient's own cognitive processes in mediating the level of activity in the pain pathway. Pain, they argued, is a highly individual and very varied experience which is influenced not only by noxious stimulation but also by the individual's expectations and anxieties, their understanding of the situation and past experience, their personality – and a host of other factors.

No longer could effective pain control be seen as a standard medical procedure applied to an isolated system within the body which would have equivalent effects regardless of who 'owned' the body in which it was situated. Melzack and Wall provided a theoretical framework for pain which demanded that a consideration of the individual patient's particular characteristics and experience be regarded as central to effective pain control.

However, accepting that the patient must be regarded as a 'whole person' whose individual pain experience must be explored if pain is to be effectively controlled, it is not necessary to accept that the patient should be given control over his/her pain treatment in the very direct manner associated with PCA. This brings us to the more specific arguments for PCA.

In her chapter Thomas explains very clearly the rationale for actually giving the patient control over the treatment of his/her pain. Control, or the perception of control, over one's situation is increasingly seen as an important influence on one's state of health. Thomas draws to our attention the beneficial effects on patients undergoing surgery of enhancing the perception of control through the use of information, cognitive strategies and behavioural control interventions. The use of PCA postoperatively obviously greatly enhances the patient's level of control. Moreover, to deny the patient as much control as possible in such circumstances may also be seen to be potentially harmful.

Thomas points out that much of the literature on the importance of personal control derives from Seligman's early work (Seligman 1975). Seligman maintained that being subjected to uncontrollable events builds up an expectation of uncontrollability which he labelled 'learned helplessness'. Subsequently it has been shown that this can adversely influence many aspects of both physical and mental health (Peterson, Maier & Seligman 1993). Whilst a state of learned help-lessness is unlikely to be established in an otherwise normal person within a relatively short postoperative period, subjecting people to markedly reduced levels of control must be seen as potentially damaging and to be avoided as far as possible.

These two types of arguments, the general and the specific, under-standably will find differing degrees of acceptance within the medical profession. Whilst it is difficult to take issue with the general proposal that the patient's individual pain experience should always be central to pain treatment, on the benefits of handing to the patient a significant amount of control over the treatment there is contradictory evidence. In her own research Thomas has demonstrated that whilst most patients benefit from PCA, some do not want to take the responsibility for their own pain control. To allocate such patients to PCA may well add to their stress. The difficulty for the doctor is not having any means of knowing who these patients are and, in the absence of more definite guidelines about identifying them, a cautious approach is to be expected. In her chapter Thomas identifies some of the variables which should be considered, and elsewhere (Thomas 1991; Thomas *et al.* 1993) has argued strongly for the development of a questionnaire which could be used to predict which patients will and will not benefit from PCA. Until such a measure is developed PCA will continue to be treated with caution by medical staff and is unlikely to fulfil its potential.

Taken at face value PCA appears to be the ultimate in patient-centred care. Consequently the reasons for its slow uptake in clinical practice are of considerable interest. The separation of general and specific arguments for PCA may allow some insight into the caution with which the technique has been treated by many medical practi-tioners in this country. Patient-centred and patient-controlled treat-ments carry different risks and perhaps require different levels of justification. In the treatment of pain a patient-centred regime benefits all patients, whereas a patient-controlled regime benefits only a proportion of them. Those who emphasize the more general arguments for PCA will be surprised and disappointed by what they will see as the medical profession's unduly cautious approach. Those who examine the more specific arguments will at least understand that caution. Thomas' chapter is important in showing where the specific arguments need strengthening and further research needs to be done. The need to distinguish between general and specific arguments for PCA may prove a valuable object lesson for those working in other areas of patient-centred care.

References

Melzack, R. & Wall, P.D. (1965) Pain mechanisms: a new theory. *Science*, **150**, 971–9.

Peterson, C., Maier, S.F. & Seligman, M.E.P. (1993) *Learned helplessness. A Theory for the Age of Personal Control.* Oxford University Press, New York.

Seligman, M.E.P. (1975) *Helplessness: On Depression, Development and Death.* Freeman, San Francisco.

Thomas, V.J. (1991) *Personality characteristics of patients and the effectiveness of patient controlled analgesia.* Unpublished PhD thesis, University of London.

Thomas, V.J., Rose, F.D., Heath, M.L. & Flory, P. (1993) A multidimensional comparison of nurse and patient controlled analgesia in the management of acute post surgical pain. *Medical Science Research*, 379–81.

III ◆ *The Context of Care: Administrative, Legal and Physical*

8 ◆ Patient-Centred Management: Patient-Centred Care Through Continuous Quality Improvement

Christopher Heginbotham

It would appear to be a truism that all health care must centre on the patient. Without patients, health services become meaningless. Yet the development of health care in the western world during the last century has emphasized professional and institutional values over those of individual patients. This has begun to change as patients have become more informed and a culture of consumerism has arisen; as health care professionals have become less paternalistic; and as health professionals and patients alike have come to realise that greater effectiveness can be achieved by a proper involvement of the patient in the process of care. Another significant influence has been the UK government's Patient's Charter initiative (DoH 1992); charter targets have now become an important lever for change. This chapter considers a number of developments in patient-centred (sometimes referred to as patient-focused) health care from the stand-point of health service management.

The principles of patient-centred management can be incorporated into various management models. One well-developed model involves a cyclical and continuous quality improvement process with four main components:

(1) organizational change and improvement;
(2) service provision with a stronger emphasis on patient involvement;
(3) review and evaluation of the effectiveness of care;
(4) organizational learning to effect further improvements.

In this chapter these critical processes are described, together with the importance of cyclical quality improvement systems geared to the steady enhancement of organizational capability. The aims and objectives of patient-centred management, and some general problems which may arise when introducing such systems, are described. Examples are then given of each of the four stages of continuous quality improvement within the improvement cycle, and from these examples a number of key lessons and suggestions for future activity are drawn.

Aims and objectives of patient-centred care

Patient-centred care is rooted in a desire to improve the quality of health service by focusing all activities on the individual patient. Patient-centred care thus aims to enhance patient autonomy within the treatment process, by developing continuous quality improvement focused on patient need, and by organizing care staff in multi-disciplinary, multitask teams which can respond quickly and flexibly to the patient. Both hospital based medical and surgical care and community services must develop a patient-focused approach, although community health services developed multidisciplinary team working earlier than many acute hospitals; for example, many psychiatric services are now organized around the multidisciplinary team often based in a locally accessible community mental health centre serving a defined geographical sector.

The primary aim of any health service is to offer the best possible care using treatments which are effective. To this can be added a number of subsidiary aims, such as managing services well, providing a good environment for staff, teaching and training health professionals, and so on. The primary aim can be further specified in terms of a number of key objectives; usually these are to:

- establish services which focus directly on the patient;
- emphasize patient satisfaction in clinical and non-clinical care;
- achieve high quality outcomes for patients;
- effect a partnership between the patient and clinical team;
- minimize hospital stay and provide care in the least intrusive environment;
- develop reliable instruments for measuring and monitoring patient care;
- understand how management affects the provision of patient-centred care;
- foster patient-centred care planning.

These objectives, if met, will of themselves generate other activity which will affect organizational management and professional inter-action, as well as teaching and education.

Getting started

A number of general problems may arise in introducing patient-centred policies. Some of these will be outlined in this section before considering in more detail the four stages of continuous quality improvement.

Many organizations want to become more patient responsive but are somehow unable to make the first steps along the road. From experience in those hospitals which have tackled patient responsive systems there appear to be three key requirements of organizational readiness. First, there must be an attitude which accepts a patient-centred approach; second, there must be a commitment to make the changes necessary to produce a patient-centred environment; and third, there must be sufficient enthusiasm to maintain the changes even when the going gets tough.

Continuous quality improvement requires a cyclical approach which recognizes the importance of change and which strives constantly for improvements without necessarily the tyranny of 'right first time'. Staff need to be engaged actively. A patient-centred approach must be reinforced continually through the many processes which go on within the organization; for example, staff remuneration should be aligned with the requirements of the quality improvement process. Often hospitals reward individual effort rather than team performance and sometimes even reward behaviours which are frankly antagonistic to a quality improvement system.

Patient-centred systems can so easily be undermined if staff do not 'own' the need for change. Especially important is team work. This will include minimization of interprofessional demarcation and rivalry, consistency in application of patient care protocols, learning from the patient, and organizational understanding of what matters to staff and patients alike. Effective care-giving often comes from integrated team work, but leadership of multidisciplinary teams continues to cause friction. This is particularly true where senior clinicians believe that leadership necessarily comes from a technological and scientific standpoint. Sometimes highly motivated, technically competent, medical staff will be critical of those qualitative systems and protocols which provide a basis for many patient-centred services. Protocols can be liberating rather than constraining, but are usually perceived as the thin end of a management wedge designed to control clinical activity, and are often seen as being for cost-cutting purposes only.

The role of management is to give strategic leadership, to act as an institutional advocate for the patients, and to suggest new ways of organizing care teams. It is not a manager's role to second guess clinical opinion. Rather managers can try to take a broader view of the organizational difficulty inherent in delivering complex multidisciplinary care under conditions of financial constraint.

Some staff perceive attempts to introduce new organizational concepts as cynical manipulation aimed at cutting expenditure. Patient-centred care is criticized as just another ruse to achieve even greater economies. With limited resources every pound must be spent as effectively as possible to patient benefit. Not to do so is unethical. Unfortunately there will always be a tension between the drive for greater economy (seen by some as cuts – especially at a time of unpopular health service reforms) and changes to the ways professional staff work which offer improved patient care. Sometimes leadership has a price (in popularity or morale) but may come to be seen eventually as both wise and far-sighted.

Most importantly the organization must establish mechanisms for enabling staff to talk to each other at all levels, to share concerns, identify problems and to generate locally acceptable solutions. Management's role is to empower – to give staff 'permission' to think the unthinkable, to criticize constructively present ways of working, and to provide a psychologically safe environment in which to argue for and promote change.

Establishing patient-centred services requires locally relevant organization and management changes. Staff involvement is crucial and multi-skilling of staff is a key component of the patient-centred approach; for example, the staff at Kingston Hospital work in teams which involve a range of disciplines, but where each member of the team is trained in a number of techniques usually appropriate to one specific discipline. Staff are then able to work across disciplines, undertaking a wide range of tasks without traditional demarcation of functions. At Central Middlesex Hospital protocol development enabled staff to learn others' jobs about which, until then, they had been largely ignorant. Lifespan NHS Trust found that to achieve a patient-focused service required involvement of *all* staff if decentralization of care was to be workable. They discovered that forming 24 hour multidisciplinary care teams added to individual skills, and care pathways improved by requiring integrated case notes and medical record systems (Wickings in NHSE 1993).

Some approaches adopted by different hospitals are described below.

(1) Where possible, patient care can be organized in semi-autonomous units with an appropriate speciality focus. There are three aspects to this:
   (a) to create self sufficient work teams with appropriate skill-mix;
   (b) to give staff local delegated control over resources and decisions affecting patient care;
   (c) to achieve improved efficiency and effectiveness by concentrating on specific condition–treatment groups (e.g. hip/ knee replacement surgery).
(2) Patient services can often be integrated more closely. Out-patient clinics can be redesigned to minimize the number of patient visits and waiting times and ensure all facilities are easily accessible. Similarly patient care can be placed as close as possible to the patients' necessary environment; for example, outreach to GP practices rather than patients travelling to the hospital.
(3) Cross-training of staff on a range of specialisms can broaden individual and thus team capability, without losing the core competencies and craft skills associated with each profession.
(4) Protocols, integrated care pathways and task critical systems can be used to manage care in multiple task oriented services. Integration

of 'demand management' and scheduling can overcome complex compartmentalized processes.

Continuous quality improvement

Systems responsive to patient need use continuous quality improvement mechanisms to develop patient-centred services and 'empowered' service users. Fig. 8.1 shows the traditional four point organizational development cycle. At the top is the stage of organizational development which includes decisions about setting or changing standards. It is at this point that a decision might be taken to develop patient-centred care. The next stage, to the right, is where the services are run with that new approach. The third stage is that of review and evaluation; and the fourth stage is that of organizational learning.

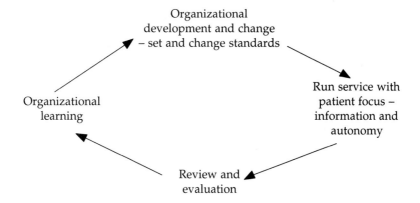

Fig. 8.1 The traditional quality cycle. Each of the four points is itself a complex of different methods and systems, of which only one example for each is given in the text.

(1) Organizational development and change – Kingston Hospital

Early in 1992 the Board of Kingston Hospital (NHS) Trust agreed to implement a 'patient-focused' approach. The decision was taken following substantial research commissioned by the Trust which showed that the hospital's service suffered many delays through inefficient scheduling, was fragmented and depersonalized, was highly centralized, had no clear focus of accountability for *total* care, and services were remote from top management (Kingston Hospital Trust 1992).

Patient-focused care is being achieved at Kingston Hospital following radical reorganization based on the following principles:

● Patient services will be placed closer to the bedside.
● Staff will be multiskilled in patient-focused teams.

- Care teams will provide a co-ordinated approach to total care.
- Each operating unit will become semi-autonomous.
- Treatment will be based on protocols or planned programmes of care.

A 'bottom up' approach was adopted. Strategic issues and whole hospital operational issues were dealt with by a leadership team, while the staff in the medical unit planned and made recommendations about their new organizational arrangements. Staff are organized in three self-sufficient teams depending upon the type of work they undertake:

(1) care givers, including nursing, psychology, radiology and other similar disciplines;
(2) administrative staff, including management and clerical staff;
(3) services associates, which includes portering and cleaning.

By using carefully crafted schedules with clearly defined patient protocols and patient pathways it is claimed that it is possible to obtain greater efficiency as well as improved quality with increased patient responsiveness. Each group participates in decisions on the extent of devolution of central services, the roles and interplay of each group, and the identification of skills necessary to carry out the agreed functions.

Implementation began by agreeing on the scope of the programme, auditing case notes and interviewing members of the medical staff, in particular the consultant body. The literature was then reviewed to identify trends and 'best practices', and an overrating method was developed. At this point the process was opened up to the input from nurses in all parts of the hospital leading to an approach which could be piloted within one part of the hospital. Amendments were made in the light of experience and protocols developed which would then be used for training and amended as appropriate. Staff and patients were surveyed for their reactions and comments. Protocol content, and the level of specification and formalities, were updated and validated against current case records.

This form of patient-focused hospital appears to have a number of benefits. Documentation time and quality benefits are high in comparison to the previous arrangements. Enormous opportunities for a detailed audit of both professional activities and outcomes and hospital organizational development are emerging rapidly. Protocols have already found a place in assisting mentoring of staff and in training and guidance for junior staff. Eventually protocols will be placed on screens and terminals at the bedside. Even in the paper version the potential for improving quality patient care and carer satisfaction has been found to be substantial.

Staff naturally fear that protocol-driven care will be used as an excuse to lower investment, reduce role differentiation and undermine professional autonomy. In practice some of these fears prove groundless. In a discussion of the role of physiotherapists in patient-focused systems, Langley (NHS Executive 1993) found that 'disguised cost cutting' had not occurred, that deskilling of staff had not happened and that jobs had actually broadened.

(2) *Running the service – information for patients: the Wennberg video disk*

To enable the patient-focused approach to work well, staff at Central Middlesex Hospital have given careful consideration to ways in which information is given to patients. This has led them to use an 'interactive video'. The concept of using video to inform patients, to offer choices and to enable patients to share decisions about treatment was first conceived and developed by a team of researchers based at Dartmouth Medical School in the USA, led by Jack Wennberg, an epidemiologist who had been working with clinicians on outcomes research in relation to the treatment of benign prostatic hypertrophy (BPH). The interactive system currently used provides men with detailed information about their prostate condition and the treatment choices available to them. The video was introduced into the UK by the King's Fund Centre in London as a development project, the aim of which is to introduce and evaluate this technology in the NHS (Darkins 1992).

The hardware for the system is a personal computer, a laser disk player, a video monitor, a video card for the PC and a printer. The software was developed at Dartmouth and enables information to be presented to patients as text, graphics, sound or full motion video. Not all patients with BPH are considered eligible to see the interactive video programme. Exclusion criteria have been devised to ensure that patients whose prostate condition is severe enough to necessitate urgent surgery, or mild enough that surgery is not considered as a suitable option, are excluded from using the video programme by their consultant. The video is seen by patients for whom the decision about treatment – whether to have surgery, whether to take medication, or whether to opt for 'watchful waiting' – is genuinely uncertain.

Each patient is introduced to the interactive video by a nurse who shows them how to use the system and helps them to enter their personal details. Patients are then left alone to see a 40 minute presentation about BPH.

Initial experience suggests that there are common misconceptions about giving information to patients – that patients will not want to know or that the issues are too complex. In practice, patients found the disk helpful and more patients than had been expected opted for 'watchful waiting' rather than surgery. BPH is not the only treatment where decisions are uncertain. Outcomes relating to the treatment for breast cancer, mildly raised blood pressure, the treatment of choice for coronary artery disease, and so on, all lend themselves to this type of presentation. Further evaluation is currently underway, and new areas for interactive systems are being considered.

The interactive video disk is one way in which patients can be given better information. Clinician time is reduced and patients obtain greater consistency in the information they receive. Patients benefit widely from the availability of information, and from having a broader understanding of their condition and possible treatment. They are thus likely to be easier to look after because they will feel more comfortable about the options open to them. Future activity is likely to use CD-ROM technology, but the time consuming aspect of the development work is in writing a sensitive patient-focused description of a condition and treatment which is at once informative but readily understood.

(3) *Review and evaluation – learning from the patient: the Picker/Commonwealth patient-centred care programme*

In 1988 at Beth Israel Hospital in Boston, Massachusetts, Dr Tom Delbanco (Cleary *et al.* 1991, 1992) decided they needed to learn more about what matters to patients. They began with a review of the literature, and compiled a primary list of those features of care that patients could evaluate and that they judged most important. These were tested in a series of focus groups with recently discharged patients and patients' families, in addition to clinical and nonclinical staff. They discovered unsurprisingly that patients' concerns fall into broadly seven categories:

- Respect for patients' values, preferences and expressed needs.
- Communication, information and education.
- Co-ordination and integration of care.
- Physical comfort and support.
- Emotional and psychological support, and alleviation of fears and anxieties.
- Involvement of family and friends (but differs between patients).
- Continuity and transition.

The importance of each of the seven categories will vary from patient to patient; for example, patients' values and preferences are not the same and this will influence their demand for information and education. Patients differ widely in their expectation of competence and efficiency, some being particularly concerned or anxious about the competence of staff, others simply relieved that their condition is to be treated. Some need physical and others emotional support; and patients vary a great deal in the extent to which they want family or friends to be involved and the extent to which they can cope with changes in ways their care is conducted. Most patients want their hospital stay to be as short as possible and for the bulk of their care to be provided in or around their home. But short stays in acute hospitals must be managed well if the care is to feel continuous rather than being a rather unpleasant short episode in an otherwise reasonable treatment arrangement.

Handling such different requirements needs understanding, and a range of ways of providing information. Some doctors are good at discussing what they are going to do for the patient but are not always good at relieving patients' fears and anxieties. This is where patient satisfaction ratings linked with factual reports can be useful. Ratings can be prescriptive, based on leading questions, but at least provide some insight to overall satisfaction. Reports, on the other hand, can generate new information about the way a service is operating; for example, a question such as 'could much of your pain have been eliminated by prompt attention from medical staff?' can evoke a range of responses and will indicate both individually and cumulatively whether staff are responding promptly and effectively to pain relief.

Other questions may be asked, such as 'Were you told about side effects?' or 'How long did the doctor spend with you?'. Such questions can then be used for action planning and to identify changes required. Focus groups of patients have also been used as a way of generating further questions for ratings and reports, and for obtaining information which might not otherwise be generated from a questionnaire format.

Using these seven categories the Beth Israel Hospital developed a more detailed patient review and evaluation, and it is now being used in a number of other hospitals in the USA (Delbanco 1992). During 1992 the questionnaire was introduced into the UK by Bruster *et al.* (1994) and used in English hospitals in a modified form relevant to the NHS. A random sample of 36 hospitals of over 200 beds was selected and a method was devised for random allocation of patients to the programme. The questions used were of two sorts: ratings and reports. Reports are seen as particularly important as these identify issues about which patients feel most concerned and enable further ratings to be developed. What emerged in the USA was that many patients are concerned not only about nonclinical but also clinical quality. Patients want to know that doctors and other clinicians are competent to undertake their care and they are capable of asking many searching and critical questions of their clinicians.

In the UK over 5000 patients were interviewed and the results show that patients' reports in response to direct questions about aspects of care differed significantly from overall ratings of care given by the same patients. Patient responses to rating satisfaction are shown in Table 8.1.

However, when asked specific questions responses were much less positive (Table 8.2). The authors conclude that satisfaction ratings must be used sparingly and where possible in conjunction with other ways of testing specific facets of patients' experience.

Regular patient evaluation systems have begun to change the way in which doctors and other clinicians perceive ways in which they give care and ways in which patients' receive that care. This has led to more patient-focused systems and ways of respecting patients' individual views of the type of care they wish to receive and the ways in which they wish to receive it.

Table 8.1 Responses to questions about patients' satisfaction. (Short list extracted from Table 1 in Bruster *et al.* 1994. Courtesy of *British Medical Journal*.)

Question	%
Very or fairly easy to understand:	
Purpose of tests	97
Results of tests	95
Explanation of operation	98
Answers to questions about operation	96
Satisfaction	
Overall rating of care excellent, very good, or good	94

Table 8.2 Responses to questions asking what happened to patients in hospital. (Short list extracted from Table 2 in Bruster *et al.* 1994. Courtesy of *British Medical Journal*.)

Response	%
No explanation from doctor about condition	16
Purpose of tests not explained	18
Not told results of tests	34
Not given explanation of operation	18
Risks and benefits of operation not explained	28
Worries and fears of operation not discussed	32
Not told about foods to eat/not eat	73
Not told about activities to do/not do	60
Not told when to resume normal activities such as returning to work	62
Not told of any warning signs to look for	70

(4) Organizational learning: The ENQUIRE system

Often organizations fail to learn the lessons of evaluation and quality systems. Many organizations make changes too quickly on immediate feedback from patients or following some form of review such as that described above. A period of organizational learning is often needed. This can come about through seminars and interactive discussions, but is perhaps best done by developing review and evaluation mechanisms which involve staff and patients in observing the service, and in reviewing the observations with other staff members.

The ENQUIRE system is an observational audit approach developed by the King's Fund College, especially but not only for community health and social care. In this method a team of staff is drawn from across the service, from all levels, from all staff disciplines, and from patients/service users. The team is then trained in observational techniques and in the use of two qualitative analytical tools: the quality matrix and the quality star. The team can also include service users or/and patients or ex-patients.

Working in pairs the team spends time with patients on wards and in facilities observing the service in action. 'Observing' includes listening, talking, hearing and seeing the service which is provided. Ward or service policies and procedures are also taken into account as context for the observations. The visiting pairs then write their observations carefully and choose for each service those which appear to be most important (usually between 15 and 30 observations are chosen). These are then analysed for content, using a number of factors, and by structure, process and outcome variables. Using this data a qualitative profile of the service is constructed.

Organizational learning is effected in two ways: by the team working together on the range of information drawn from specific facilities, which is collated and analysed; and by feedback of action plans from the team to all the wards and facilities visited. Action plans have to be 'owned' and accepted by the staff and patients on the wards. This leads to discussion about the process or observation, the significance of the observations and the proposed actions. The importance of generating outcome data emerges strongly from the process.

The ENQUIRE system has been used in a wide variety of health and social services locations, largely in acute and continuing care for people with mental illnesses, learning disabilities and disability associated with old age. Predominant problems include the staff time needed for effective training, observation and feedback, and clinicians' reluctance to accept even methodologically rigorous *qualitative* information as of the same value as quasi-objective 'scientific' data, even if much of that is based on unvalidated experimental designs. The advantages of ENQUIRE include a focus on the qualitative aspects of care that matter most to patients, the achievement of staff involvement and ownership, and the generation of new standards which staff and patients believe to be appropriate.

An example of ENQUIRE in practice is provided by staff in Mid-Glamorgan Social Services Department. Staff in Mid-Glamorgan undertook an initial series of observational visits to a range of community mental health services. This led to a set of revised standards for hospital wards, day services and residential care. For brevity only a selection of the standards referring to hospital wards are given (Table 8.3). The implementation of these standards can be observed on second and subsequent 'passes' when standards can be checked, amended or enhanced.

Most of the standards which emerged were of a non-clinical nature but expressed the feelings of both observers and patients about their most pressing concerns on the first set of visits. Further 'passes' will consider whether these standards are being met, and may then delve further into clinical issues when some of the 'hygiene' factors have been met.

Table 8.3 Hospital wards in Mid-Glamorgan.

The service currently provides care to the following standards

(1) Hospital staff will make themselves accessible to patients and treat them with courtesy and respect.
(2) Hospital staff will provide patients with as much information as possible appropriate to the individual's care and wellbeing.
(3) Hospital staff will endeavour to create a relaxed and informal atmosphere in their units while maintaining a safe and secure environment for the patients. Rules and regulations should be kept to the minimum necessary to maintain personal safety.
(4) Managers will be aware of staff morale in hospital units and identify and improve issues that reduce staff morale.
(5) Patient documentation will be of a high standard and reviewed regularly.

The service will endeavour to meet the following standards

(6) Facilities for patients to make snacks and hot drinks will be provided on wards and units.
(7) Staff will be given the necessary counselling skills to maintain telephone counselling services.
(8) Patients who have identified rehabilitation needs will be reintroduced into the community in a planned and phased way.
(9) Hospital staff and managers have a responsibility to ensure that patients' privacy is respected at all times. This will be reflected both in staff attitudes and the physical provision of suitable furnishing and fitments.
(10) The choice and frequency of meals will reflect the expressed preferences of the patients.

Staff empowerment through the use of care protocols

Although organizational change to achieve a patient responsive environment can be threatening, it can also be empowering if handled correctly. Many managers and clinicians now accept the wisdom of delegation with proper monitoring, and the devolution of budgetary control as far down the organization as possible. Unhappily this does not occur as often as might be expected. By delegation of responsibility to front line staff (those who actually spend or commit resources), or to immediate supervisors (who are responsible for overseeing the use of resources), staff can be given much stronger feelings of control and thus of satisfaction with their job.

Increasing interest in the use of clinical protocols and patient pathways has developed during the last few years. Protocols are being developed in order to ensure sensible resource allocation where purchaser health authorities wish to delineate more clearly which patients get what sort of care. In these cases protocols must be developed between the purchaser authority and the clinicians providing care.

Involving staff in developing care protocols (within which they offer collaborative care plans to patients) can be a liberating experience rather than one of constraint. Protocols ensure consistency and regularity in the process of care. They speed up some aspects of the delivery of care but need not diminish the opportunity for creativity amongst consultant clinicians, nor take away a consultant's ability to go outside the protocol if he or she feels it is appropriate (although clinicians have to have a good reason for amending protocols in particular instances).

Protocols assist in the development of more efficient and quality sensitive services. At Central Middlesex and Kingston Hospitals protocols are used as a basis for all care in the patient-focused wards. The protocols act as a template against which to measure clinical care and as a regular check list on key quality items in the patient's treatment. Protocols vary in their complexity and there is still some concern about whether protocols should be linked to 'rationing'. Integrating protocols into the wider work of the hospital, especially where patients with a range of different conditions are being nursed on one ward, will need further work, and will require careful discussion between purchasers and providers. More importantly, protocols should not be allowed to drive out creativity. At worst protocols would simply enshrine practice at a particular date; at best they provide a clear framework leading to consistency and efficiency whilst providing a baseline for further clinical development.

Protocols and integrated care pathways (ICPs) offer a way of defining key procedural features of a patient's care and the standards which apply at each stage. Protocols cannot contain all detailed policies, practice notes and professional standards; those are an accepted underpinning of all clinical care. Protocols need to achieve a careful balance of detail and generality relevant to the particular situation. In Riverside Mental Health Trust, for example, ICPs have been developed for adult acute and forensic admission wards. A 'top–down' approach defines the broad scope and sets clear procedures for the service; a bottom-up approach defines the pathway for each patient within the overall protocol. Not only does the ICP provide a structure and process check list, but it ensures consistency, gives a system for audit and, in Riverside Mental Health Trust, is used as the core (or backbone) of the Trust's integrated quality strategy.

Protocols provide a benchmark against which to test alternative treatments, and a framework which is known to provide safe and therapeutic care. Protocols and patient recovery pathways can be established by mutual discussion amongst the multidisciplinary team (including consultant clinicians and, where necessary, managers from both the purchaser and provider), and can offer a way of ensuring that allocated resources are used most effectively to meet the demands of the maximum number of patients. As Orchard (NHSE 1993) (St Helier NHS Trust) has pointed out, consultants are the only medical members of the care team with continuous contact over long periods of time. Consultants are thus fundamental to the success of patient-centred care, but only through input to an integrated, self directed care team.

Protocols or pathways have been found to offer a template on which to build a consistent service understood by all. They are not a strait-jacket but rather a framework which reduces errors and allows the flowering of creativity. Rather than having to remember every stage of the treatment process the clinician can be empowered to develop appropriate alternatives, freed from the necessity to remember detailed management requirements for each patient.

Some common concerns and difficulties

Many barriers exist to effective patient-centred care. These include resource levels and resource allocation procedures, new technology, potential problems of litigation, medico-legal difficulties (especially in the USA), the need to change organizational cultures, reaction from senior or influential clinicians, conservatism amongst staff generally, and a lack of drive from senior management to see that change is made. Patient-centred management is seen by some as simply the 'flavour of the month', an imported idea which does nothing more than indicate that doctors in North America have recently discovered patients! Conversely it is seen as a genuine concern by clinicians, as well as hospital managers, of the need to focus services more directly towards patients.

A number of issues remain to be considered. The development of quality measures with patient satisfaction ratings and reports may raise expectations which cannot be fulfilled, though regular consumer evaluation will indicate ways in which the service can be changed and improved. Doctors and other clinicians must be sensitive to the con-sumers' views and be prepared to amend their clinical practice. It is still unclear whether the development of protocols will be seen by some, notably young go-ahead clinicians, as threatening their clinical freedom and ability to innovate.

A further concern is that patient-responsive management systems are just another way of masking cuts or developing efficiencies which are not in the long term best interests of patients. The managers most active in developing these systems deny that this is their intent. Even so, patient-centred systems may be most easily applied where there is rapid throughput of patients requiring one or two specific procedures such as cataract removal or hip replacement. The patient-centred model may be less attractive for patients with complex or difficult problems, whether these are medical or surgical. That does not deny the importance of focusing on the individual patient and ensuring that the staffing of the ward is both efficient and effective. If, though, pro-tocols are necessary to achieve the efficiencies required, these will be of less effect where there are patients with a wide range of different conditions, or similar conditions but of varying complexity and co-morbidity.

Finally there is the problem of getting started for those hospitals wishing to develop this type of approach. It is time consuming for managers and clinicians alike, requires considerable negotiation with staff interests and can be threatening to both clinical and nonclinical staff. Any change must be handled sensitively and must be justified. Removing demarcation barriers will be difficult, particularly where these are rooted in professional training. The pilot projects undertaken so far thus provide extremely helpful experience in the difficulties of implementation.

Conclusions

In summary, patient-centred management should be seeking to achieve the key points shown in Table 8.4. Developing patient-centred and patient-responsive management demands an integration of organizational development and professional clinical practice. One must not drive out the other; nor is a woolly compromise sufficient. But there is tension between management directed change and the craft aspects of individual clinical care, and this tension must be recognized. Rather than an uneasy compromise, a model of synergy is required, drawing on and valuing both approaches to improving patient care and a recognition that each approach has strengths as well as weaknesses.

Good clinical work is based on long experience of helping patients. Management must recognize the 'craft' aspects of clinical practice, especially nursing, and must recognize that organizational or structural solutions are not, by themselves, the answer. Clinicians must recognize that managers are not interested simplistically in structural solutions, and that patient-centred models are not promoted merely as a way of achieving financial savings. Efficiency and economy are important but must be balanced by attention to clinical best practice, effectiveness of interventions, staff morale, safety and patient satisfaction.

Table 8.4 Future prospects for patient-centred care.

- Establish health care environments which are receptive to protocols and patient involvement.
- Set up collaborative planning – a useful strategic device for involving patients and professional players.
- Develop 'least able to communicate' advocacy for those who have difficulty speaking out.
- Challenge vested interests by asking 'who is the customer?'.
- Share information and communication.
- Provide patients' access to protocols and records.
- Strive for organizational implication.
- Use patient information and involvement on service design, and place premium on patient views.
- Give patients choice in treatments provided.

Protocol development is a positive driver for improved care and resources. By demonstrating that a minimum practice model is essential, the resources have to be found to meet it. Achieving consistency in procedure and standards reduces 'error' or 'failure' costs, improves morale, reduces sickness rates, raises patient satisfaction and encourages team creativity and innovation. That at least is what we should be striving for.

Health service management will need to develop a culture of consumerism which involves patients at all stages and recognizes that it is the patients' needs which are paramount, and that systems must support the patients rather than patients being seen as incidental to the hospital's function. All systems, be they clinical or nonclinical, must place a premium on improving outcomes as defined by the patients' views.

References

Bruster, S., Jarman, B., Bosanquet, N., Weston, D., Evans, R. & Delbanco, T.L. (1994) National survey of hospital patients. *British Medical Journal*, **309**, 1542–9.

Cleary, P.D., Egman-Levitan, S., McMullen, W. & Delbanco, T.L. (1992) The relationship between reported problems and patient summary evaluations of hospital care. *Quality Review Bulletin*, February, 53.

Cleary, P.D., Edgman-Levitan, S., Roberts, M., Moloney, T.W., McMullen, W., Walker, J.D. & Delbanco, T.L. (1991) Patients evaluate their hospital care: a national survey. *Health Affairs*, **10**, 254–67.

Darkins, A. (1992) *Helping patients make decisions* (unpublished). King's Fund College, London.

Delbanco, T.L. (1992) Enriching the doctor–patient relationship inviting the patient's perspective. *Annals of Internal Medicine*, **116**, 414–18.

DoH (1992) *The Patient's Charter*. HMSO, London.

Kingston Hospital Trust (1992) *The Patient Focused Approach.* Prepared by J. Langan for a seminar at the King's Fund College, London, December.

Mid-Glamorgan County Council Social Services Department (1992) *Quality Assurance Through Observation of Service Delivery – a Practical Approach.* Mid-Glamorgan County Council, Cardiff.

NHSE (1993) Conference on patient focused care. Incorporating *The Therapist Perspective* (J. Langley); *The Nursing Perspective* (G. Morgan); *The Medical Perspective* (R. Orchard); *The Researchers Perspective* (I. Wickings). HMSO, London.

Richards, H., Heginbotham, C. (1992) *Enquire: Quality Assurance Through Observation of Service Delivery.* A workbook, 2nd edn. King's Fund College, London.

Reading guide

There is now a large literature on quality improvement in health care, though surprisingly little rigorous academic work on patient satisfaction and standards. A good introductory text is Øvretveit (1992) which provides a wide ranging, practical workbook for health care quality initiatives. More challenging is a publication by the National Quality Care Forum in the USA (NQCF 1992) in which a series of authors and respondents explore the latest work in the USA and offer a compact theoretical position. For the more ambitious reader, or one with sufficient time, the standard quality management textbooks are: Berwick *et al.* (1990), Crosby (1983), Deming (1986), Juran (1989) and Watton (1986). All of these authors have written many papers, one of the best being Berwick (1989).

Berwick, D. (1989) Continuous improvement as an ideal in health care. *New England Journal of Medicine*, **320**(1), 53–6.

Berwick, D.M., Godfrey, A.D. & Roessner, J. (1990) *Curing Health Care.* Jossey-Bass, San Francisco.

Crosby, P.B. (1983) *Quality without Tears: the Art of Hassle-free Management.* American Library, New York.

Deming, W.E. (1986) *Out of the Crisis.* Massachusetts Institute of Technology, Cambridge, Massachusetts.

Juran, J.M. (1989) *Juran on Planning for Quality.* Free Press, New York.

NQCF (1992) *Bridging the Gap between Theory and Practice – Exploring Continuous Quality Improvement.* National Quality Care Forum, Washington.

Øvretveit, J. (1992) *Health Service Quality – An Introduction to Quality Methods for Health Services.* Blackwell Science, Oxford.

Watton, M. (1986) *The Deming Management Method.* Dodd, Mead, New York.

Commentary on Chapter 8

David W. Millard

This commentary takes a somewhat different starting point from that of the chapter, to which it is nevertheless a response. Rather than the *processes* of quality management, it deals primarily with the personnel responsible for this – and, indeed, other – managerial tasks in health care delivery. Particularly, it is interested in the structural relationships between some of the main actors involved.

Empirically defined social groups are the principal tool of sociological analysis. The sociological study of professionalism during recent decades has typically been in terms of the politicians, the bureaucrats and the professionals. Generally, these have been seen as being engaged in a kind of three-cornered battle for the control of the welfare agencies, and studies within this genre have tended to emerge with conclusions consonant with Bernard Shaw's wisecrack that all professions are a conspiracy against the laity. For our present purposes, I suggest we need to add to these the managers and the users of health care services. There is of course nothing especially inviolable about these groups: they are defined in this way solely because I wish to suggest it is useful to do so.

Parenthetically, a comment may be made about the choice here and in the chapter of the term user. I am mildly astonished that the conference whence these texts originated, and where the philosophers took very seriously the implications of the ordinary usages of language, should have undertaken no explicit criticism of the word patient. Every time we employ it we must subliminally remind ourselves of its etymology: one who suffers, the passive recipient of whatever treatment anyone else chooses to hand out. Its antonym is agent; surely a term conveying much better, if imprecisely, the ideology implicit in the title of this book. A number of other terms are conveniently employed to circumvent the limitations of the word patient. In social work client is commonplace, while consumer (as in Heginbotham's chapter) and even customer occur in welfare contexts where economic or management considerations are in mind. All these, and others, have senses that are capable of misleading. Currently I think the least objectionable and the broadest in its reference is user, and this has the added advantage of being the word widely adopted by a variety of self-initiating groups of those to whom it applies.

On the other hand, there exists a reality which only one or two contributors have explicitly acknowledged: that the experience of serious illness causes most people of whatever age to behave for a limited period as children behave. A convenient term for such age-inappropriate behaviour is regression. No doubt because of reservations specifically surrounding Freudian analysis, the vocabulary of psychodynamics and the rich body of theory and practice associated with it have remained unremarked. Nevertheless, both the Rogerian ideas called upon by Hope in Chapter 11, and the pastoral psychology of Campbell employed by Titchen in Chapter 12, have some indebtedness to this school of thought. The point here is that regression and user empowerment represent to some extent contradictory motions in the relationship between the helped and the helpers.

The potential contribution of the users to maintaining quality standards in health care varies across a wide spectrum which must eventually reach a boundary (e.g. with the unconscious patient); hence the theory of regarding doctors, for example, as purchasers of the services on their patients' behalf and its implementation in general practice fundholding. For the user, caveat emptor has unavoidable limitations! Heginbotham is surely right to stress the importance of handing more information to the users, as in the Wennberg interactive video experiment, but we must be sensitive to the range of application of this approach.

But to return to my main theme: persons in each of the social groups mentioned earlier may share many common characteristics which differentiate them from members of the other groups – a broadly shared system of concepts, knowledge and skills, a broadly shared set of values and beliefs, a broadly similar process of induction into group membership and of rules which permit continued membership or mandate expulsion, and so on – in short, a common culture.

Of course individuals may migrate from one group to another: professionals may become politicians, bureaucrats may become managers as, indeed, within the health service many have done. But poachers turning gamekeeper tend to become especially exacting gamekeepers; proselytes are said to be particularly devout. There is much sociological evidence that people's behaviour is shaped more strongly by the social group within which they find themselves than it is by their individual qualities. Thus, it is proper to consider group characteristics.

Among a multitude of such characteristics, social scientists would typically distinguish power and authority. Elaborate analyses of these concepts are available in the literature. Briefly, power is the capacity of the holder to obtain the compliance of others, whether or not in the face of opposition. It rather easily transforms itself into right and the corresponding obedience into duty. Authority arises out of social relationships, within which it requires legitimizing by those over whom it is exercised (i.e. consent). Power and authority may co-exist, but certainly need not do so; for example, unauthorized power is to be observed in tyrannies, or actions may be authorized which those responsible are powerless to carry out.

A crucial issue in considering the delivery of patient-centred care is the analysis of the power and authority relationships existing between the five groups identified above. How do these matters stand currently, and how should they be in order to optimize a patient-centred style of health care? These are wide-ranging questions, and it is not possible to offer a comprehensive response here. Three related themes are offered as examples; each has some reference to the chapter.

Implications of quality management

Heginbotham is very properly concerned to trace the implications for managers and clinicians of quality management; significantly, one of his emphases is staff (i.e. not user) empowerment. Given the changes now crystallizing out of the NHS and Community Care Act 1990, we cannot avoid comparing present-day British health care delivery to that of 1948 when the arrangements most closely approximated the Beveridge ideal. In what senses do staff require empowerment?

Who, then, have been the gainers and who the losers? The following are crude impressions; some evidence could be adduced, but space here does not allow. It appears that the politicians have become slightly less powerful; this is probably true of Westminster politicians and certainly of local politicians. Bureaucrats (often administrators in welfare terminology) have experienced a swingeing loss of power and accompanying reduction in status. The power of the professionals has probably remained practically unaltered, although there have probably been some shifts within the group (nurses and social workers more powerful, doctors less). The managerial class has arrived from nowhere (in practice, many former bureaucrats and a fairly small proportion of professionals have become managers) and become substantially powerful. Finally, the users have perhaps become marginally more powerful.

We may note that the rise of managers is a universal phenomenon of western societies in the 20th century, accelerating after 1945. It began in manufacturing and commerce with a separation between ownership and management (compare the 19th century woolmaster – typically, owner and manager of his mill), in part as a consequence of the increasing size and complexity of enterprises, and has now spread to welfare enterprises. The concept of the managerial revolution, so-called after a book of that title by J. Burnham in 1941, which mistakenly predicted that at macrosociological level a managerial class would supersede the old capitalists – does not cut much ice nowadays. But I propose the changes outlined above constitute a managerial reformation in the welfare services – that is, a re-forming of the managers' power structures, beliefs, relationships and so forth. Within western cultures this may turn out to have been as radical as the reformation in 16th century religion.

Not a new ideology

Is the patient-centred ideology new? I think not. Politicians have believed throughout that they were authorized to enact an ideology in the user's best interests; the rhetoric has been persistently 'Patients first'. The change has been in what that phrase denotes. In 1948 the anxiety against which users were to be protected was the financial burden of sickness – hence, the universal service free at the point of delivery and the ultimate evolution of concepts like the social wage. The policy costs included an out-of-control and inefficient bureaucracy. By 1990, the anxieties against which the users had to be protected were to do with access (waiting lists, regional inequalities, etc.) – hence, the internal market, the managerial reformation, and the other power adjustments noted above. However, the user's anxieties were confounded by those of the politicians – the alarm at the escalating financial burden (itself driven by scientific advance, demographic changes and shifts in social expectations) which conflicts with other objectives which they have in the nation's or their party's interests. The fear to which Heginbotham refers is very real among many in the professional and user groups: that some of what passes for patient-centred care is motivated by the politicians' cost-cutting agenda.

Intergroup relationships

I think we need greater clarity about what energizes these intergroup relationships. Obviously this includes money, and some social scientists have argued that the only true power is economic. But money is not the only motivator, nor is it necessarily the most influential; and nor is it the only medium of social exchange. For example, when we speak of user empowerment this does not generally extend to financial control over welfare services.

Particularly in health and welfare organizations, personal relationships matter hugely. Heginbotham notes in passing that '... staff remuneration should be aligned with the requirements of the quality improvement process'. But traditionally, one of the rewards and sources of job-satisfaction for the professionals and, to a lesser extent, the bureaucrats has been the gratitude of the users. Warm and close, though of course properly bounded, relationships infuse the giving and receiving of this type of service at every point. However, managers by virtue of their structural position within the organization are almost entirely insulated from rewards of this type. So if this brief comment has any hypothesis of its own to develop, it would be to ask whether the fact that the most powerful group of actors is cut off from the most powerful set of mediators in the intergroup process does not mean that the managerial reformation is at high risk of acting to the detriment of patient-centred care. Perhaps the managerial class will be able to develop a culture which in some way protects it from the effects of isolation from these sources of affirmation. If not, it may fail to deliver quality – not through any personal inadequacy on the part of those concerned, but by virtue of the structure and dynamics of the health care organization.

9 ◆ Patients First: the Role of Rights

Jonathan Montgomery

Rights are increasingly used as powerful slogans by those who wish to enhance the power of patients. Pressure groups, the government and international bodies have all produced statements of what they see as good practice expressed in terms of rights; for example, three of the ten rights set out in Cancerlink's *Declaration of rights of people with cancer* are directly concerned with the relationships between patients and health professionals:

'(3) ... to know I have cancer, to be told in a sensitive manner and to share in all decision-making about my treatment and care in honest informative discussions with relevant specialists and other health professionals.
(4) ... to be fully informed about treatment options and to have explained to me the benefits, side effects and risks of any treatment.
(6) ... to a second opinion, to refuse treatment or to use complementary therapies without prejudice to continued medical support.'

The present UK government's Patient's Charter champions a number of patients' rights in the NHS, and will be considered in more detail below. At a European level, a resolution of 19 January 1984 committed the European Parliament to the production of a European Charter of Patients' Rights. Although as yet no such document has emerged from the institutions of the European Community, a draft European Convention on Bioethics has emerged from the Council of Europe's Human Rights machinery (Byk 1993; Council of Europe 1994).

The language of rights thus has an important place in the rhetoric of patient empowerment. In general, however, debate has proceeded without subjecting the concept of a right to detailed scrutiny. This chapter seeks to appraise the value of 'rights' as a tool for promoting patient-centred care. It discusses how far English health care law can be said to accept patients' rights and what it might look like if it did. The strengths and weaknesses of adopting a rights-based approach to patient-centred care are examined.

The idea of rights

The concept of a 'right' became one of the key ideas in modern political philosophy in response to the difficulties presented by the widespread acceptance that some form of utilitarianism presented the best foundation for concepts of justice (Hart 1983). Utilitarians believe that action is morally justified if its net consequence is to increase pleasure and decrease pain. Such a doctrine aggregates total benefits and harms and disregards the fact that individuals do not experience those harms and benefits equally. Thus it could appear just to kill a healthy person in order to harvest their kidneys, liver, heart, lungs and corneas for redistribution, if doing this would increase the aggregate welfare of the human race.

Rights can provide a counter-balance to the excesses of such consequentialist theories in two important ways. First, they can be used to ensure that all individuals are treated with equal concern and respect (Dworkin 1977, 1985). This means that the distribution of benefits must be taken into account as well as their aggregate (Scanlon 1977). Second, rights can be used to identify certain components of an individual's wellbeing that are so fundamental that they may not merely be traded off to secure collective benefits (Dworkin 1977). This is not necessarily to say that rights can never be overridden, but only by unusually strong claims, perhaps only by claims based on similarly fundamental rights which are in conflict.

Important insights into the nature of rights have also emerged from analysis of the law. The 18th century legal philosopher, Jeremy Bentham, saw the key to understanding the concept of a right in terms of its effect in placing obligations on others. He contended that, as enforceable obligations can only exist within a legal system, it was nonsense to conceive of rights except in a legal context. Appeals to 'natural rights' were merely an empty rhetorical device aimed to confer a spurious dignity on the claims being made. However, he argued that within a legal system the concept of a right was extremely useful (Hart 1982).

Modern jurisprudential analysis has shown how rights-talk can be seen as a particular way of describing the relationships between people. It is thought that people have rights when obligations are imposed on others in order to promote the interests of the right-holder (Raz 1986). Duties that are justified not by reference to an individual's interests, but by some collective public good, do not reflect rights. This approach is known as the interest theory of rights.

Understanding the nature of the obligations that constitute rights can tell us a great deal about the status of that right-holder. Rights based on interests alone are compatible with paternalism, in that they can be used to formalize the duties to care for individual patients without enhancing those patients' control over their care. Orthodox medical ethics, based on the professional duties of nonmaleficence, beneficence, autonomy and justice can be recast in terms of rights with little difficulty.

Some thinkers have gone further and adopted 'choice' or 'will' theories of rights. These require not only that obligations serve the interests of the right-holder, but also that the right-holder is able to decide how and when to exercise their rights (Hart 1982, 1983). For those who wish to increase the power of patients, the choice theory of rights is more attractive because it emphasizes the ability of right-holders to control the position of others.

It can be seen from this discussion that the idea that patients have, or should have, rights offers an important framework for promoting patient-centred care. A strong scheme of patients' rights would have a number of characteristics. First, it would place the patient at the core of their relationship with those who look after them by defining professional responsibilities in terms of the interests of patients, not the expression of normative values created by the professions. Second, it would give power to patients by giving them control over the exercise of their rights. If empowering patients is the aim, then only rights that maximize choice would contribute to that objective. Third, conferring rights on to patients would imply that their choices and needs would prevail over general policy considerations. Rights provide constraints on cost-benefit calculations in the interests of individuals and prevent certain types of trade-off. Thus the rights of patients could not be sacrificed to the common good. Finally, rights must be enforceable if they are to have any real existence. Even if it makes sense to talk about rights in a purely moral sense, a strong scheme of patients' rights would need to enable patients to vindicate their rights in some way. In the next section I will consider how far English law incorporates effective rights for patients.

Current English law

The Patient's Charter boldly asserts that NHS patients possess ten rights. Six cover access to health care: the right to receive it on the basis of clinical need rather than ability to pay, to be registered with a GP (and therefore receive primary care), to receive emergency care, to be referred to a consultant or for a second opinion, to information on the quality of local services (according to measures chosen by the government or NHS rather than the patient), and to be admitted for inpatient treatment within two years of being placed on a waiting list by a consultant. Three cover the position of the patient once they are receiving care: the right to a clear explanation of proposed treatment (including alternatives and risks), to have access to records (which are guaranteed to be confidential), and to be permitted to choose whether or not to be involved in research or training. The final charter right covers enforceability: the right to have complaints investigated and to receive a full and prompt written reply.

None of these rights really stands up to scrutiny, however. The mechanisms for enforcement are weak; NHS complaints procedures are widely regarded as unsatisfactory (DoH 1994; Chapter 14 in this book). Attempts to claim access to health care have shown how the interests of individual patients do not prevail over other considerations (Montgomery 1994a). The courts have said that they will not get involved in resource allocation decisions because these raise political rather than legal concerns. Nor will they interfere with clinicians' decisions about the priority of particular patients or refusals to admit to waiting lists, unless perhaps they are made on an illegal basis such as race or gender. Nor, as a matter of principle, will they order doctors to treat patients in a manner contrary to their clinical judgment. In the light of this reluctance to enforce the promised rights of access, it should be recognized that they are not really rights at all.

The weakness of English law's commitment to patients' rights can perhaps be best seen in relation to the right to be informed about your care. The control of information is a key factor in defining the balance of power between patients and those caring for them. The degree of information required to be given to patients before their consent is regarded as valid is one aspect of the distribution of information. However, the English law of consent fails to recognize patients' rights in any significant sense (Montgomery 1992a). There is a promising basic legal principle that, where a legally valid consent can be obtained, care cannot be given to a patient without consent. However, English law does not require that such a consent should be informed other than in 'broad terms', so that it is clear that the patient has agreed to the procedure that is to be performed rather than a different one altogether (*Chatterton* v. *Gerson* 1980). To ensure that patients can actually exercise control over their care, it is necessary to ensure that they possess sufficient information to weigh up their options. In English law this is not seen as an issue about consent, but as part of the general duty of health professionals to act properly (i.e. according to their own professional standards). Thus a claim that a patient was not told enough can only succeed if the professional who counselled them was negligent. This can only be proved if it is possible to show that all responsible professionals in the field would have given a fuller explanation (*Sidaway* v. *Bethlem RHG* 1985). While this hands-off approach to a fundamental issue of patients' rights has been widely criticized (e.g. Kennedy 1991), attempts by the lower judiciary to scrutinize professional practice more closely have been suppressed by the Court of Appeal (Montgomery 1988).

Another aspect of information control is access to health records. In this context English law has conferred rights upon patients. Under the Access to Health Records Act 1990, patients are entitled to see their own health records and to correct inaccuracies. They are also entitled to receive an explanation of unintelligible parts of the record, a provision that should help shed light on the mysterious jargon of health care. The Access to Health Records Act goes a considerable way to reduce the power of health professionals to control patients by withholding information from them, and the Act's long-term importance in opening up a secretive professional culture should not be underestimated. However, in some areas of controversy, such as the right to know of a poor prognosis demanded by Cancerlink, the Act will do little to enhance patients' rights. This is because the rights that it creates are limited by the fact that access can be denied where the health professional believes that disclosure would be likely to cause serious harm to the patient's health. This allows parts of the records to be left out of material given to the patient. While the need to protect patients from some information may be conceded, the fact that it is health professionals who control the application of the exception undermines the strength of the patient's rights.

Further, in English law the duty of confidence that health professionals owe cannot be said to be based on the rights of patients. Confidentiality is conceived by the courts as existing in the public interest in efficient health care, not as a result of patients' interest to privacy. It follows that confidentiality is readily outweighed in the public interest because there is no patients' right at stake to give any priority to the principle.

In short, when the existing state of English law is examined, it is clear that it does not provide a strong scheme of patients' rights. In the key area of control of information, the patient's position is weak. While there is a clear requirement that consent to treatment is obtained, the standards of 'informed' consent are set by the professions, not for them. Access to health care records provides an example of a genuine right (established by Parliament rather than the courts). However, even here the degree of patient control is undermined by the fact that health professionals may limit the exercise of the right of access where they believe that the patient's health would be affected. The rights of patients to ask for particular types of care, or even to receive care at all, are weak.

This reluctance to build English health care law on the concept of rights is deliberate, not accidental. In general, the English judiciary, and until recently the English legislature, has been particularly reluctant to compromise the clinical freedom of the medical profession (Montgomery 1989). Moves towards greater constraint on medical freedom can clearly be seen in respect of the statutory licensing of embryo research and some infertility treatment (Montgomery 1991). The terms of service of general medical practitioners have become more specifically and rigidly defined by the government (Jacob 1991). However, these moves towards closer regulation of medical practice should not be seen as increases in patients' rights in the strong sense. Although medical power is reduced, patient power is not thereby increased. The Mental Health Act 1983 introduced an important rights-based framework (Unsworth 1987). However, it too deals primarily with restraining medical power, rather than empowering a group of patients whose contested capacity to exercise choice constitutes the very problem that has to be solved.

Strengths and weaknesses of the rights approach

Some lawyers argue that medical law is essentially an area of human rights law, and therefore bemoan the failure of English law to adopt a rights-based approach (e.g. Kennedy 1991). It is important, therefore, to evaluate the strengths and weaknesses of rights as a tool to further patient-centred care. A move towards patients' rights would involve a number of fundamental changes of attitude, some of which may be less attractive than others. This section discusses some of the implications of concentrating on rights, in terms of the restructuring of the relationship between patients and their carers.

Amongst the legal rights that do exist, are the information rights created by the Opticians Act 1989. Under that Act, UK opticians are required to supply information about care. When they perform a sight test, they must provide the patient with a written prescription stating what is necessary to correct their sight. On the face of it, this is an example of a right to information that will provide a small step towards a legal guarantee that consent to treatment is truly informed.

In context, however, the objective of this provision can be seen to be to ensure that patients' power as economic agents is preserved. Normally, it is very difficult for patients to assess the value of professional services because they do not know what they need to buy. By ensuring that they will be armed with the specifications that they need, the impact of this lack of knowledge is reduced. The provisions of the Act also seek to ensure that this purchasing power will be real by prohibiting opticians from requiring patients to promise to buy glasses or contact lenses from them as a condition for testing. In cases where the NHS is to pay for such appliances, the same market forces are unleashed by providing patients with vouchers that they can use to pay for them. (The relevant law is to be found in the Opticians Act 1989, s.26, the Sight Testing (Examination and Prescription) (No 2) Regulations 1989 (SI 1989 No. 1230) and the NHS (Optical Charges and Payments) Regulations 1989 (SI 1989 No. 296) Part IV.)

The thrust of these provisions is that patient choice can be enhanced by dividing the process of diagnosis from that of treatment. Thus a patient can shop around for the best deal on treatment, being able to compare like with like. This use of rights is directly linked with an understanding of patients as nothing more than economic actors. The introduction of patients' rights is, in fact, being used to subject opticians to the discipline of the economic market. It is possible that the whole patients' rights movement is so closely linked to consumerism, that the attractiveness of rights matches that of consumerism.

The essence of consumerism is that consumers should get what they want, not what producers choose to offer them. It follows that the greater the control that patients exercise, the more restricted clinical expertise becomes. While the real extent of clinical freedom in a large bureaucratic health service should be examined carefully, in theory the law leaves considerable scope to practitioners to follow their professional opinions. The only formal rights of conscientious objection are to be found in the area of reproductive medicine (Abortion Act 1967, s4; Human Fertilisation and Embryology Act 1990, s.38). Nevertheless, for doctors at least, the inability of patients to force them to provide any particular pattern of care leaves clinical judgment unrestricted.

Health professionals are thus permitted to deny patients access to health services which have been accepted as appropriate by society, under the guise of clinical freedom. This privileges professional values over those of patients and gives professionals power at the expense of patients. The law is rather less favourable to nurses because it reinforces the subordination of their professional freedom to that of doctors (Montgomery 1992b). However, nurses remain privileged in relation to their patients.

To disturb the current pattern of deference to professional judgement by introducing extensive patients' rights would challenge a number of fundamental characteristics of the professions' self-image. The assumption that patients can exercise choice implies that the issues can be understood by nonexperts, and denies the notion of an exclusive, scientific knowledge base. It also devalues the need for skills of interpretation, learnt only in practice. Over time the recognition of patients' rights could alter the very nature of professional practice by suppressing the personal and professional values of practitioners. Whether professionals think that care is appropriate would become less important than whether patients want it.

A further concern arises from the possibility that rights are essentially reductionist, reducing the complex social reality of patient-centred care to a narrow range of entitlements. The language of rights has no place for virtues such as compassion, altruism and sacrifice. Indeed, it could be argued that to adopt a rights-based approach to health care could destroy the very virtues on which it has been traditionally founded. Some see rights as unnecessarily antagonistic, promoting confrontation rather than partnership by emphasizing the entitlement of one party at the expense of the voluntary service of the other. These are highly significant features of a rights-based system when the position of health professionals is considered. Patients' rights may devalue the contribution of health professionals, both in terms of their expertise and in terms of the values their vocations enshrine. If these characteristics are thought to be the very qualities that enhance patient-centred care, then rights could prove profoundly counter-productive.

These points illustrate that rights are about power. Deciding what rights to create is in large part a process of determining who should hold what power. Professions, and probably in particular the medical profession, have traditionally wielded considerable power over their patterns of work (Johnson 1972). This has been achieved partly because of the vulnerable position of patients and it is likely that this degree of occupational control could not be sustained in the face of a strong system of patients' rights. Thus, it is probably true that a commitment to patients' rights entails abandoning some aspects of traditional professionalism. It is also important to note that debates about rights inevitably involve power struggles between professions. Health care rights could be little more than a mechanism for transferring power from health professionals to lawyers in courts (Hope 1991; Rose 1985).

If no benefits are seen by patients, then a move towards rights would be no more than a victory for law over medicine.

Conclusions – a right role for rights?

This chapter has shown how rights can be employed to emphasize the importance of individuals over general values. It has argued that English health care law has shown little interest in rights, although some steps have been taken to define and curtail the power of the health professions. It has considered some of the implications of adopting a rights-based strategy to patient-centred care and has suggested that it would involve subjecting the comfortable privileges of the health professions to the wishes of patients. Refocusing power away from the health professionals, and towards the patient, is a key element in promoting patient-centred care but it is not without its dangers. It is now necessary to grasp the nettle, and consider how power should be allocated, and whether, notwithstanding the difficulties, rights can indeed foster the primacy of patients.

The focus of the chapter has been on the position of patients in relation to the professionals looking after them. Issues in relation to access to care have received only brief treatment (for more, see Montgomery 1992c). There the redistribution of power entailed by the introduction of rights would be away from politicians and managers, rather than clinicians. However, the key problem is common to both groups: how can the complexity of a patient's position be captured in a system of rights, which must by its nature be generally defined, without undermining the possibility of care being tailored to patients' needs? This is the difficulty of reconciling the indeterminacy of health care with the legitimate claims of patients.

The solution can be illustrated by two proposals for reform in relation to the doctrine of consent: proposals for new provisions for living wills and for informed consent. I have put forward detailed cases for these changes elsewhere (Montgomery 1992c, 1994b). Here they serve to show how rights can improve the position of patients without falling foul of the difficulties spelt out earlier in the chapter.

The need for consent before treatment is lawful is an example of a right that provides a constraint on professional paternalism. It ensures a basic degree of patient control over care, forbidding treatment that the patient does not want. However, it is a right that is not universally conferred on patients by English law; it is only held by those who are competent to consent. While in principle it makes sense to restrict this right to give or withhold consent to those who are competent to exercise rational choice, the way in which they are categorized leaves much to be desired. This has proved particularly problematic in relation to adolescents (Montgomery 1994c) and to the terminally ill. Health professionals can remove patients' rights by declaring them to be no longer competent to decide (Kennedy 1991). Thus, while in principle patients are entitled to be left to die, doctors can nullify the effect of that right by a finding of incompetence.

One way around this is to guarantee that patients' earlier wishes are respected, strengthening their right to die. Considerable, and proper, disquiet is felt by the health professions at giving such advance directives or living wills binding force. The principal worry is that a binding living will would force the health professionals to do something inappropriate and remove their discretion to tailor their care to the patient's present needs (as they see them). This is precisely the problem of rigidity and if it cannot be overcome, then rights strategies are unattractive. It is, however, possible to provide for more flexibility, whilst still enhancing patient choice.

Advance directives could be given legal force, without making them operate as rigid constraints on clinical decisions. The law could impose a prima facie obligation on health professionals to refrain from treating patients in breach of the terms of an advance directive. Prima facie obligations are not absolute, because they can be outweighed by other considerations. The right of the patient to decide in advance to die would therefore act as a weighty 'trump' that could only be overridden for very good reasons, reasons that should be specified by the law. The function of the legal right would be to require health professionals to respect the wishes of the patient unless the reasons for disregarding them were overwhelming. It would not be enough that the health professionals disapproved of the patient's decision.

A second area where reform is necessary is that of informed consent. Here too, the use of patient's rights as a restraint, or brake, upon health care decisions, rather than an insurmountable barrier, also provides the way forward. A law that made a consent invalid unless it has been fully informed would fail to reflect the fact that there may sometimes be valid reasons for withholding information. This can be seen in North American law, where a 'therapeutic privilege' to keep information secret in order to protect patients has developed alongside strong doctrines of informed consent, and judges have felt the need to find technical arguments to undermine doctrinal strictness (Robertson 1981).

However, if the legal principles of informed consent can be established as presumptions, so that their breach gives rise to a prima facie but not unchallengeable case of malpractice, the problem of rigidity can be reduced. Thus the law could require health professionals to disclose all the information that a prudent patient would want, unless the patient had either expressly declined to exercise their right to know it or there were compelling reasons to believe that disclosure would cause serious harm to the patient's health. The law would then specify the tests to be applied in deciding what to tell a patient. The sophistication of this approach would be enhanced if a code of practice were to elaborate these concepts further. Failure to adhere to the code would be evidence of malpractice, but health professionals would be permitted to escape liability by justifying their decision to depart from its guidance.

These two examples show how the problems of rights–strategies can be overcome. An unthinking acceptance of patients' rights is dangerous, because introducing the wrong sort of rights would be as damaging to patients as continuing to ignore their rights altogether. However, with that caveat, rights offer an important strategy for promoting patient-centred care. A fundamental review of health care law is needed, with a view to providing a coherent and comprehensive framework of health rights (Montgomery 1992c).

Reading guide

For an introduction to the theory of rights, see Freeden (1991). Some important contributions to the primary literature on the philosophy of rights are collected in Waldron (1984). Discussion of rights in the legal system can be found in Dworkin (1977, 1985), Hart (1983) and Raz (1986). Many of the essays in Kennedy (1991) examine health care law from a rights perspective. Montgomery (1989) argues that English law generally supports medical paternalism rather than patients' rights, and Montgomery (1992c) proposes a scheme of health rights for English law.

References

Byk, C. (1993) The European Convention on bioethics. *Journal of Medical Ethics*, **19**, 13–16.

Chatterton v. Gerson (1980) 1 BMLR 80.

Council of Europe (1994) Draft European Convention of Bioethics (Council of Europe, Strasbourg). *Bulletin of Medical Ethics*, **99**, 19–24.

DoH (1994) *Being Heard.* Report of a review committee on NHS complaints procedures (the Wilson Committee). Department of Health, London.

Dworkin, R. (1977) *Taking Rights Seriously.* Duckworth, London.

Dworkin, R. (1985) *A Matter of Principle.* Oxford University Press, Oxford.

Freeden, M. (1991) *Rights.* Open University Press, Milton Keynes.

Hart, H.L.A. (1982) *Essays on Bentham.* Oxford University Press, Oxford.

Hart, H.L.A. (1983) *Essays in Jurisprudence and Philosophy.* Oxford University Press, Oxford.

Hope, R.A. (1991) The birth of medical law. *Oxford Journal of Legal Studies*, **11**(2), 247–53.

Jacob, J. (1991) Lawyers go to hospital. *Public Law*, 255–81.

Johnson, T. (1972) *Professions and Power.* Macmillan, London.

Kennedy, I. (1991) *Treat Me Right.* Oxford University Press, Oxford.

Montgomery, J. (1988) Power/knowledge/consent: medical decision-making. *Modern Law Review*, **51**, 245–51.

Montgomery, J. (1989) Medicine, accountability and professionalism. *Journal of Law and Society*, **16**, 319–39.

Montgomery, J. (1991) Rights, restraints and pragmatism: the Human Fertilisation and Embryology Act 1991. *Modern Law Review*, **54**, 524–34.

Montgomery, J. (1992a) The contribution of law towards raising standards of consent. In *Consent to health treatment and research: differing perspectives* (ed. P. Alderson, pp. 37–46). Institute of Education, University of London.

Montgomery, J. (1992b) Doctors' handmaidens: the legal contribution. In: *Law, Health and Medical Regulation* (S. McVeigh & S. Wheeler), pp. 141-68. Dartmouth, Aldershot.

Montgomery, J. (1992c) Rights to health and health care. In:*The Welfare of Citizens* (ed. A. Coote), pp. 83–107. Rivers Oram, London.

Montgomery, J. (1994a) Legal issues in prenatal diagnosis. In: *Prenatal Diagnosis: The Human Side* (eds L. Abramsky & J. Chapple), pp. 23–36. Chapman & Hall, London.

Montgomery, J. (1994b) Power over death: the final sting. In: *Deathrites: Law and Ethics at the Ending of Life* (eds D. Morgan & R. Lee), pp. 37–53. Routledge, London.

Montgomery, J. (1994c) The retreat from Gillick. In: *Children's Decisions in Health Care and Research* (eds P. Alderson & B. Mayall), pp. 7–14. Institute of Education, University of London.

Raz, J. (1986) *The Morality of Freedom.* Oxford University Press, Oxford.

Robertson, G. (1981) Informal consent to medical treatment. *Law Quarterly Review*, **97**, 102–26.

Rose, N. (1985) Unreasonable rights: mental illness and the limits of the law. *Journal of Law and Society*, **12**, 199–218.

Scanlon, T.M. (1977) Rights, goals and fairness. In: *Theories of Rights* (ed. J. Waldron, 1984). Oxford University Press, Oxford.

Sidaway v. *Bethlem RGH* (1985) 1 BMLR 132.

Unsworth, C. (1987) *The Politics of Mental Health Legislation.* Oxford University Press, Oxford.

Waldron, J. (ed.) (1984) *Theories of Rights.* Oxford University Press, Oxford.

Commentary on Chapter 9

John Devereux

Montgomery's chapter has convincingly demonstrated that patients' rights in England are more rhetoric than reality. He has provided us with a thorough coverage of the issues involved. The plain fact, as Montgomery demonstrates, is that such rights are *not* well entrenched in English law, despite the bold statement of patients' rights contained in the Patient's Charter.

I would like to consider two issues, particularly as these are illuminated by the law in other countries. The first is the distinction between the exercise of a right, and that right's continued existence. In the USA where, as Montgomery has noted, patients enjoy greater right to information about proposed treatments and their risks, academics have pointed out that some patients do not use the information with which they are provided by medical practitioners. Those who do assimilate the information may use it for purposes other than deciding whether to consent or refuse consent to treatment. One group of researchers identified four different uses made of information provided, only one of which was clearly information sought and used for decision making about treatments (Lidz *et al.* 1982). Given that patients are not using detailed information about their treatments, it might be questioned whether there is any sense in continuing to enforce their right to receive such information; that is to say, is there a reason to continue to recognize the existence of a right to information?

Arguably there is a reason: in short, just because someone fails to exercise a right, it is no reason to extinguish that right. In law, a waiver of a right is binding only on the particular occasion that the waiver refers to. Waiving a right today is not prejudicial to any future exercise of a right. Common sense also tends towards this conclusion. So in the UK, generally speaking, a person is free to travel within the UK (or, with valid travel documents, overseas). We would say that people enjoy the right to freedom of movement. We would not normally suggest, just because someone has lived in the same village for the last 40 years without availing himself of his right to travel, that when he decides to celebrate his 40th birthday by travelling to London, he should be denied the right to travel simply because he has never travelled before. So it should be with patients' rights. A failure to exercise patients' rights, even by many people, should not cause the demise of such rights.

The second issue I should like to address is why patients' rights have not developed as fully in the UK as in other English speaking countries. Although I am unable to point to empirical evidence, I suspect that the fact that treatment under the NHS is largely offered free of charge, is a cogent reason for the lack of a broad-based movement for greater patient rights. It may simply be a question of patients not looking a gift horse in the mouth. If a patient is offered, free of charge, treatment which is medically efficacious, why should she complain about a lack of information or a threat to her autonomy? I suspect that patients would be more vociferous if they had to pay something towards their cost of treatment.

It is interesting to note that currently in Australia all but the poorest patients have to pay for their treatment, and are then reimbursed about 85% of the doctor's fee by the government. There is a safety net to ensure that no one pays above a set amount of money per year in medical expenses. Beyond this amount, the government pays all medical bills. The very poor pay nothing – the government is directly charged. All this operates within a system in which GPs are self-employed. Patients are not obliged to join the list of any practitioner. They may attend one practice one day and another in the same region on the next.

The High Court in Australia has recently broken with UK authorities in holding that a doctor has a duty to disclose such information about a treatment (including risks) as a reasonable patient would expect, or as the doctor knows or ought to know that this patient expects (Rogers & Whittaker 1992). Montgomery points out that, over time, the recognition of patients' rights could alter the very nature of medicine. The decision of the High Court of Australia is a good example of this principle. The High Court of Australia suggested that, as the provision of information about a proposed treatment did not involve the exercise of peculiarly medical skills, the test of whether a medical skill was exercised negligently or not (i.e. did it conform with what a reasonable body of medical practitioners would do?) did not apply to the disclosure of information. It would come as a surprise to many doctors that their disclosure of information about technical medical procedures to their patients was not part of their medical skills.

The health care complaints legislation in a number of Australian states has been revamped. It is unclear whether the operation of the Medicare system in Australia has contributed to the increase in patients' rights there. Nonetheless, it is suggested that patients who were forced to pay for their treatment, even if such sums would subsequently be reimbursed, would be likely to be more critical of the provision of health care.

Similar developments can be seen in New Zealand. The health care system is currently in a state of flux, but the system is moving to a more 'user-pays' philosophy, so that all but the poorest will contribute something towards health care costs. At the same time, New Zealand has enacted in its Bill of Rights Act 1990 a provision which has been expressed to be without precedent in human rights documents (Austin 1992). Section 11 of that Act provides that everyone has the right to refuse to undergo any medical treatment. Perhaps greater or clearer patients' rights are the quid pro quo of charging for health care. Already the courts are whittling down the width of such a right in New Zealand (S 1992). Given the reluctance of political parties to commit Britain to a written constitution, the enactment of a similar guarantee of one of the patients' rights seems unlikely.

The issue of patients' rights may ultimately be seen as a means of enforcing patient-centred care.

References

Austin, G. (1992) Righting a child's right to refuse medical treatment. *Otago Law Review*, 7(4), 578.

Lidz, C.W., Meisel, A., Holden, J.L. & Munetz, M.R. (1982) Informed consent and the structure of medical care. *Making Health Care Decisions*. United States Government Publishing Office, Washington.

Rogers & Whittaker (1992) *Australian Law Journal Reports*, **67**, 47. S (1992) *New Zealand Law Reports*, **1**, 363.

10 ◆ The Planetree Model Hospital Project

Steven F. Horowitz

'Healing the soul is as important as healing the body' (Hippocrates)

The Planetree concept was created in San Francisco in 1978 by Angelica Thieriot in response to her own unpleasant but medically correct hospital experience. Initially designed as an educational resource centre, the project expanded to become a 13 bed medical surgical inpatient unit within California Pacific Hospital in 1981. The basic objective of the experiment was to create a more humanistic, patient-oriented, hospital-based environment that more thoroughly addressed the emotional and educational needs of the patient and family without compromising standard medical therapy.

Within the domain of patient-centred care, the Planetree concept falls largely within the realm of patient empowerment, with services provided to allow patient and family to become more independent, better educated health care consumers. The experimental unit in San Francisco received a great deal of media exposure, attracting attention at a time when the patient-centred care movement began to take hold as a concept, but there were few dedicated inpatient units yet available for study as models. Initial surveys in San Francisco suggested nurses and physicians found the Planetree environment to be a more satisfying workplace compared to control units, and patients were generally more content on the Planetree Unit.

The name Planetree derives from the plane tree, or common sycamore, under which Hippocrates taught. On the basis of widespread interest in the first Planetree Unit, and a desire to test out the feasibility of the project under a variety of conditions, Planetree subsequently extended its network to include four additional model hospital sites. Three sites were located on the west coast of the USA, and one site in the north-east. Beth Israel Medical Center in New York City was selected as a model site to assess the viability of the Planetree concept in a more difficult inner-city, urban environment. In addition to the model units, more than 20 affiliates have since been enrolled, including European sites in Poole, England, and Trondheim, Norway.

The Beth Israel Medical Center is a large teaching hospital located on the lower east side of New York City. This area of Manhattan is densely populated and is traditionally called the melting-pot of New York, consisting of numerous ethnically diverse populations. This diversity is reflected within the hospital, where translators are available for over

40 languages, including four Chinese dialects. In addition to treating economically solvent, well-insured patients from the five boroughs of the city, significant homeless and drug addicted populations are served as well. Patients are equally divided between private and public ('service') cases. The hospital includes the Bernstein Institute for medical and psychiatric treatment of drug dependency and related illnesses, containing the largest methadone maintenance programme in the nation.

The Medical Center is a teaching affiliate of the Albert Einstein College of Medicine and is associated with several community health centres, including a large Hispanic clinic, a Japanese medical centre, and a health service largely dedicated to the needs of the orthodox Jewish community. In its aggregate, the Medical Center contains more than 1300 inpatient beds, and has the fourth largest number of patient discharges in the USA. The Samuels Planetree Unit is a renovated general medical floor consisting of 34 beds (two private and 14 two-bedded rooms, together with a four-bed cardiac care stepdown unit).

The objective of the physical remodelling of Planetree was to create a residential rather than institutional sensibility to the floor. The renovation of the Unit included several innovations that had symbolic as well as aesthetic importance. Primary among these was the elimination of the traditional nursing station (Figs. 10.1 and 10.2), felt to be a psychological barrier between patient and staff. The four foot high separation was replaced by a waist-high semicircular desk, allowing free access by staff and patients on three sides. Additional corridor space was opened up to family and patients, with access restrictions only within offices, medication rooms, and staff lounges.

Corridor lighting was offset so that patients lying on stretchers would not look directly into bright fluorescent lights. Speakers were placed at regular intervals to allow for continuous playing of soothing music. Art work was carefully selected to present calming yet upbeat colours and themes. Pictures with potentially negative symbolism – such as cold, isolated landscapes, dark colours, or scenes with empty chairs or swings – were avoided.

The family room was transformed from a relatively sterile environment lined with chairs and tables into a comfortable and warm setting with private alcoves, book shelves, sofas, reclining seats, and table lamps. The room was equipped with donated books, art materials, games and puzzles, and a television set with accessible VCR and taped movies. The family room also became the focal point of various Planetree sponsored events, including staff lectures to patients and family members, holiday parties, picnics and concerts. Every effort was made to convey thoughtfulness through the design of the family room in an effort to avoid the impression that the room was assembled as an afterthought (Figs. 10.3 and 10.4).

Rooms and bathrooms were redone with designer-selected, aesthetically pleasing floors and accommodation. The unit was constructed as a collaboration between designers and engineers from both San

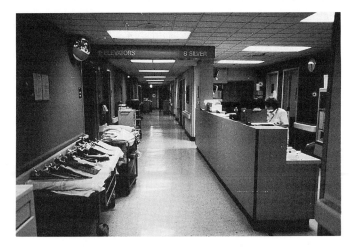

Fig. 10.1 A traditional nursing station.

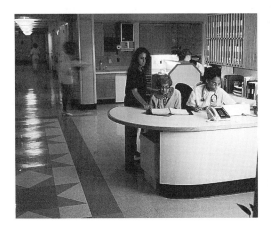

Fig. 10.2 The same nursing station, after renovation work, providing a more patient-friendly atmosphere.

Francisco and New York City. During the design phase, the colour patterns originally selected by the San Francisco designers were universally rejected by the staff on the east coast. Less vibrant, sedate colours were felt to be more appropriate in the frenetic New York environment, while vibrant colours had more appeal in the more 'laid-back' atmosphere of California and Oregon. Wood furnishings and shelves replaced metal wherever possible, and construction materials were carefully selected for their appearance as well as for durability and low cost.

The latter two attributes have clearly become dominant influences on materials selected for urban hospital construction and renovation. Every attempt was made to service these requirements without seriously disrupting the aesthetic objectives of the floor. A continuous dialogue was required between designers, architects and hospital

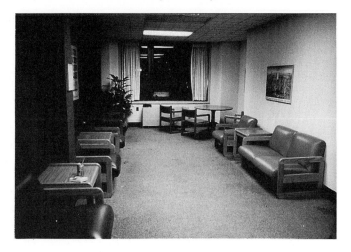

Fig. 10.3 A traditional family room.

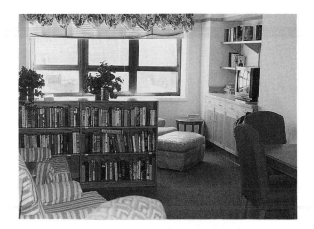

Fig. 10.4 The same family room after renovation, designed to give a patient-oriented environment.

engineers. In most instances satisfactory compromises could be achieved, but this proved to be a labour- and time-intensive task. This undoubtedly prolonged the planning phase of our unit, but was deemed necessary to avoid the pitfalls of standard hospital construction, which, although maximally efficient, often produced compromises that inadvertently conveyed a diminished concern for the patient.

As with many other facets of the creation and maintenance of the Planetree model, a chronic requirement of the project has been the omnipresent need to refocus attention on the needs of patient and family. This focus is often lost behind closed administrative doors as decisions are made based, understandably, on bottom-line considerations and expediency. In addition, decisions must take into account the needs of special interest groups, such as physicians, nurses, administrators, unions and community boards, and too little feedback comes from patient interviews, surveys or focus groups.

Representatives from the Julliard School of Music perform regularly on the Unit, providing live chamber music concerts and short plays for the patients. A small kitchen was added to the floor to allow for preparation of favourite foods and 24-hour availability of snacks. A full-time nutritionist uses the kitchen for teaching demonstrations and for baking cookies and cakes, a welcome event for both patients and staff, and an opportunity to replace the standard antiseptic hospital smells with something a bit friendlier and more familiar.

An arts coordinator provides materials and supervision for patients and family members who wish to express themselves through drawings and paintings, which are then displayed in the family room. A story-teller regularly visits the floor and talks to groups of patients as well as bed-bound individuals within their rooms.

These, and other similarly designed programmes, such as healing touch and massage, create a lighter, less oppressive hospital atmosphere that allows both patient and family member to reframe the inpatient experience. Many patients respond poorly to verbal reassurances alone but are deeply touched by music, art or familiar foods. During the initial Julliard School performance no call lights went on during the hour and a half concert, which is virtually unheard of in a high acuity ward with a 95% occupancy rate.

The full therapeutic value of these ancillary services, as a complement to traditional medical practice within a hospital setting, is unknown. Patients, health care workers and administrators (especially those responsible for the financial status of the hospital) may have markedly different perspectives on what constitutes an amenity versus what is a legitimately valuable medical service. An elderly person who is isolated and rarely leaves home may find that a television set represents a familiar companion rather than an amenity.

An illustrative clinical example of the approach to the patient on Planetree is a 33-year-old man with multiple hospital admissions for Crohn's disease. The patient had already been hospitalized for more than two weeks, was actively bleeding from two ileostomies, continued to have pain, and had just clotted a femoral intravenous catheter, which was his last available venous access. At this point, the patient was advised of the need for urgent surgical placement of the intravenous line in order to maintain his pain medications and blood transfusions. The patient refused because he had become infected in the past from a similar catheter. The patient was depressed, fearful and withdrawn, while the medical staff simultaneously labelled him as a problem patient and withdrew from him out of frustration with their inability to successfully treat his acute episode with standard medical therapy.

At this juncture, the nurses organized a rotation to provide brief personal contact hourly, simply to keep the patient emotionally connected with the staff. A psychologist assigned to the Unit spent some additional time talking with the patient, and the medical staff were made aware of their own withdrawal from the patient. The physicians were encouraged to resume 'caring' for the patient in the truest sense of the word, and drop their judgement of the patient as uncooperative.

The day this intervention started, the patient's pain became more manageable, improvement began without intravenous medication, and he required no further blood transfusions. While potentially coincidental, this and other similar observations on the Planetree floor have served to enhance respect and awareness of the mind–body–spirit relationship, which is often inadvertently ignored within the hospital environment. It has also served as the stimulus for discussion as to how to craft the next generation of clinical outcome studies to evaluate the impact of these 'soft' adjunct interventions.

The physician's credo of 'cure rarely, relieve suffering often, and comfort always' commonly rings hollow in the modern, high-tech hospital environment. Cure, often at any cost, has become the paradigm of the western physician, even though cure can realistically be accomplished in the minority of patients. The emotional withdrawal of the physician from the patient when cure cannot be obtained has been recognized, but remains commonplace. The concepts of relief of suffering and provision of comfort are relatively labour-intensive, and the latter essentially nonreimbursable within the current health care structure. The idea that caring should be restored as an endpoint in itself was not considered to be a highly significant issue in the recent American health care debate.

Depression and anxiety may be present in most hospitalized patients, who are understandably fearful in their new setting, removed from the familiarity of home and the reassurance and nurturing of friends and family. This is exaggerated by an impersonal hospital experience that extends from a sterile, institutional architecture to health care workers who may interact only by taking something from the patient (e.g. a history, electrocardiogram or blood sample), or doing something to the patient (e.g. a surgical procedure or an invasive diagnostic test). Often, very little time is spent relating to the patient as a fellow human being. This role may be taken up successfully by physician, nurse or ancillary worker, but the ongoing emphasis on efficiency aimed at shortening the length of stay, provides little time for any paid hospital staff to fill this role.

On the Planetree Unit, every effort is taken to afford nurses more time at the bedside, and other staff personnel and volunteers attempt to create at least one trusting relationship with the patient. In addition, there are open visiting hours and a care partner programme designed to maximize the emotional support of the patient. Although not yet studied on the Planetree Unit, it is logical to assume that relief of anxiety will ultimately diminish requirements for pharmacologic sedation and, as in the case of the young man with Crohn's disease, may ameliorate some anxiety-related disease exacerbations.

A major role of Planetree, therefore, is to serve as the patient's advocate for all decisions that affect the physical and functional operation of the Unit, both bedside and within the board room. For this patient advocacy to be effective, a primary refocusing of attention on all the needs of the patient is required, with replacement of the patient into the number one position of priority within the health care system.

Acknowledgements

The author wishes to thank Deborah L. Matza, RN, MPH, Director of Nursing, Planetree, Beth Israel Medical Center, and Arthur E. Blank, PhD, Senior Health Services Researcher, Beth Israel Medical Center, for their review of the manuscript.

The Samuels Planetree Model Hospital Unit was named for a gift from the Fan Fox and Leslie R. Samuels Foundation. Other grants were provided by the United Hospital Fund and Citibank.

Reading guide

Bandura, A. (1977) Self-efficacy: toward a unifying theory of behavioural change. *Psychological Review*, **84**(2), 191–215.

Bartlett, E.E. (1992) Patient-centered health care: desideratum for medical care reform. *Patient Education and Counselling*, **19**, 237–9.

Belkin, L. (1992) Hospital study tests benefits of giving comfort with care. *The New York Times*, 26 September.

Blank, A.E., Horowitz, S.F. & Matza, D.L. (1995) Quality with a human face? The Samuels Planetree Model Hospital unit. *The Joint Commission Journal of Quality Approvement*, **21**(6), 289–99.

Cassell, E.J. (1991) *The Nature of Suffering and the Goals of Medicine*. Oxford University Press, New York.

Chase, S., Wright, J.H. & Ragade, R. (1981) Decision making in an interdisciplinary team. *Behavioural Science*, **26**, 206–15.

Cleary, P.D. *et al.* (1991) Patients evaluate their hospital care: a national survey. *Health Affairs*, 254–67.

Cleary, P.D. *et al.* (1992) The relationship between reported problems and patient summary evaluations of hospital care. *Quality Review Bulletin*, **18**, 52–9.

Davis, K. *et al.* (1990) *Health Care Cost Containment*. Johns Hopkins University Press, Baltimore.

Devine, E.C. (1992) Effects of psychoeducational care with adult surgical patients: a theory-probing meta-analysis of intervention studies. In: *Meta-Analysis for Explanation: A Casebook* (eds I.T.D. Cook *et al.*). Russell Sage, New York.

Dossey, L. (1993) *Healing Words: The Power of Prayer and The Practice of Medicine*. Harper, San Francisco.

Goffman, E. (1961) *Asylums: Essays on the Social Situation of Mental Patients and Other Inmates*. Anchor Books, Garden City, New Jersey.

Hall, J.A., Milburn, M.A. & Epstein, A. (1933) A causal model of health status and satisfaction with medical care. *Medical Care*, **19**, 84–94.

Hirokawa, R.Y. & Johnston D.D. (1989) Toward a general theory of group decision making; development of an integrated model. *Small Group Behaviour*, **20**(4), 500–23.

Kaplan, S.H., Greenfield, S. & Ware, J. (1989) Assessing the effects of physician–patient interactions on the outcomes of chronic disease. *Medical Care*, **27**(3), suppl. 2110–27.

Lathrop, J.P. (1993) *Restructuring Health Care: The Patient Focused Paradigm.* Jossey-Bass, San Francisco.

Moloney, T.W. & Pau, B. (1993) Rebuilding public trust and confidence. In: *Through the Patient's Eyes: Understanding and Promoting Patient-Centered Care* (eds M. Gerteis *et al.*). Jossey-Bass, San Francisco.

Orr, R. (1987) A new design for modern health care: the Planetree project. *World Hospitals: The Official Journal of the International Hospital Foundation*, **23**(3 & 4), 38–40.

Reiser, S.J. (1993) The era of the patient: using the experience of illness in shaping the missions of health care. *Journal of American Medical Association*, **269**, 1012–17.

Sahney, V.K. & Warden, G.L. (1991) The quest for quality and productivity in health services. *Frontiers of Health Services Management*, **7**(4), 2–10.

Sherer, J.L. (1993) Putting patients first: hospitals work to define patient-centered care. *Hospitals*, 5 February, 14–18.

Sokal, R.R. & Rohlf, F.J. (1995) *Biometry*, 3rd edn. W.H. Freeman, New York.

Townsend, M.B. (1993) Patient-focused care: is it for your hospital? *Nursing Management*, **24**, 74–80.

Vogel, D.P. Patient-focused care. *American Journal of Hospital Pharmacology*, **50**, 2321–9.

Wakefield, D.S. *et al.* Understanding patient-centered care in the context of total quality management and continuous quality improvement. *Joint Commission in Quality Improvement*, **20**, 152–61.

Commentary on Chapter 10

Trevor Martin

As an architect working on hospital design over the past two decades, I have witnessed the growing concern over future patterns of health care design. Recent changes in diagnostic services and surgical practice, and especially the increasing trend towards day surgery and out-patient care, have made it necessary to reassess the basic organization of hospital buildings. At the same time, rapid advances in technology have dictated that greater flexibility in the design of health care buildings is essential if we hope to respond efficiently to future needs. Certainly, the trend towards patient-centred care has had a radical impact on the design approach. Architects have been able to respond positively to client bodies who seek not only to implement major organizational changes in their hospitals but who, at last, recognize the important part that the built environment can have in the healing process.

Consider a typical NHS hospital. It is large and has been built piecemeal over a period of time. Traditionally it has been organized along departmental lines, with the result that patients and staff have had to cover substantial distances within the hospital in order to use equipment or obtain specialized services. Often their journey has been made difficult and stressful by poor signage systems, harsh lighting and unpleasant cooking/cleaning odours. Frequently they are surrounded by materials and finishes which are more suitable for the operating theatre than the recovery ward.

In 1992, as architect in charge of phase 2 for the West Dorset General Hospital NHS Trust (one of the first 'patient focus' hospitals to be designed in the UK), I organized a study tour of hospitals in the USA, in order to experience at first hand the latest design thinking and practice in patient-centred care. Our study group consisted of architects, a health planner, a medical consultant and an NHS chief executive. Our itinerary included a tour of the 25-bed medical/surgical unit at San Jose Medical Centre and the Planetree Health Resource Centre. We were given a guided tour of the unit by Robin Orr (then National Director of Model Hospital Projects) who explained the Planetree approach to hospital design.

The architect, Marc Schweitzer, had adopted a three-pronged approach to the project:

(1) He gained first-hand experience of the patient's perspective by staying overnight in the hospital.
(2) He consulted user groups, i.e. patients, carers, nurses, doctors, dietitians and housekeeping staff, in order to establish their needs.
(3) Finally, he met with the appropriate officials to review the specifications.

The result of this collaborative approach was readily apparent in the San Jose Unit. As in Horowitz's unit, described in the chapter, the nurses' station, traditionally so imposing with its high counter, had been rethought. The physical barrier between staff and patients had been removed to encourage better communication between patients and staff. The counter had been replaced by an open planned space at the hub of the unit where patients were able to read their medical charts and discuss their treatment with staff in comfortable surroundings furnished with low tables and informal seating.

Monotonous colour schemes and institutional grid layouts which dull the senses had been abandoned. Instead, non-standard soft furnishings and a variety of different bedroom layouts had been designed to emphasize each patient's individuality. Further scope for personalizing bedrooms was provided by shelving and bulletin boards for the patient's use. This humanized health care design approach extended to the smallest details, including the hand-painted ceramic tile room numbers. The patient's perspective from his hospital bed had been considered and special care given to the ceiling mouldings and border details. Soft carpeting had been used to reduce noise levels on the unit and to reinforce the domestic rather than institutional ambience.

The lighting had been carefully designed for patient-centred care. In the bedrooms, patients were given control and choice, with adjustable lighting on dimmer switches as well as task lighting for reading and writing. All the fixtures were decorative and residential in appearance. In the public areas, warm, indirect lighting had the effect of shortening the hospital corridors. In the patients' lounge, lighting was used to create intimate seating arrangements.

A special feature of the Planetree model is the on-unit kitchen which is open to patients and visitors 24 hours a day. Apart from the commercial grade dishwasher specified to meet hygiene regulations, the kitchen recalled the comforts of home, with familiar fittings and cabinets. It also provided an extra place for socializing while preparing a snack. A dietitian gave demonstrations and advice on the preparation of special diets. The aroma of fresh baking on the ward was an added sensory bonus.

The clean lines and uncluttered look of the Planetree Unit had been achieved by designing suitable storage facilities. Inventories of equipment and supplies were taken and future needs projected before calculating areas. Staff training sessions were provided. As a result, when equipment was not in use it was not in sight.

From an architectural point of view, the carefully restored Victorian, domestic building which houses the Planetree Health Resource Centre, immediately conveyed a message of warm welcome and open access to information. Books, cassettes, video tapes and health classes were all on offer inside. So too, was information on medical diagnoses, treatments and options. The Centre was equipped to provide computerized searches of the latest developments in medicine, as well as information on standard and experimental treatment. By encouraging patients to become more informed and to participate in health care decisions which directly affect them, the Planetree approach aims to alleviate stressful emotions such as fear and despair which are often symptomatic of ignorance and lack of control. At San Jose, the polished wooden bookshelves, comfortable seating and warm lighting provided a personalized health care setting where the patient's physical and aesthetic comfort were given priority.

The Planetree model tackles a number of important issues in relation to patient-centred care. Most importantly it has questioned and continues to question our preconceptions of what a hospital is and what a health care system should provide for the patient. Planetree champions the case for patients to learn more about their own health and for patients to actively participate in and to demand much more from the health care system and in turn from health care professionals. The

Planetree programme has shown that this can work successfully on a small scale in the USA, but the question remains – can it work on a larger scale and indeed does it translate readily into the health care system that currently exists in the UK?

By its limited size and nature the Planetree Unit at San Jose can only hope to tackle some of the issues raised in the patient-centred care debate. Without doubt the Planetree model has successfully answered a number of critical questions that need to be answered on a more general level within our health care system. However, I believe that the major advances in fostering the ideals of patient-centred care will come from the way our health care system is reorganized and the way we view health generally in terms of preventative measures. We need to review advances in the latest technology available to us and to consider how best we can incorporate them in our designs to bring services closer to the patient's bedside. The technology currently available to us enables services to be decentralized within our acute hospitals and within our communities. Already this is happening in larger scale developments being carried out under the Planetree programme and in a number of hospitals which are currently being designed along patient-centred lines in this country.

It remains to be seen whether the more far reaching organizational changes and the larger scale developments currently being effected are successful in tackling the broader issues of patient-centred care. Let us hope that they do not lose sight of what has been achieved by the Planetree programme and that the spirit of what the founder, Angelica Thieriot, set out to achieve can be sustained.

IV ◆ *Education and Training*

11 ◆ Teaching Practice Skills to Medical Students

Tony Hope

The central aims of the Oxford Practice Skills Project are to develop and evaluate a teaching programme for clinical medical students in practice skills – that is the combination of ethics, communication skills and the law. In this model of teaching, these three elements are integrated into a series of clinically centred seminars.

The practice skills approach has both theoretical and practical origins. At the theoretical level, Fulford's work on the way in which the patient's values and experience of illness permeate even such apparently 'factual' and 'objective' concepts as diagnosis leads directly to the practice skills concept (see Chapter 1 and Reading guide).

At the practical level the course developed initially from my teaching experience. I used a weekly seminar with students attached to general (internal) medicine to encourage discussion of those issues which the students thought important but for which there was no other opportunity for discussion. By the end of the first term it struck me that the issues which students chose were issues of communication. By the end of the second term I had changed my mind: the issues were not primarily about communication, they were about ethics. By the end of the third term I realized that both views were correct. Ethics and communication skills could not be separated.

Consider, for example, breaking bad news. Within the first few weeks of working on the wards most students had accompanied a patient undergoing a diagnostic test – endoscopy and biopsy of a tumour, for example. It happened frequently that the student was the first person the patient would ask for information on what had been found. What should the student say? The situation raises ethical questions, about the role of students, for example, but also about a whole range of issues to do with test results that predict a poor prognosis. How much should be said? When? When could it be right to tell a relative more than the patient? Should the doctors and nurses communicate more hope than they themselves feel? These ethical questions cannot be separated, however, from issues of communication. What and how the patient should be told raises issues both of ethics and communication skills at the same time.

This close connection between ethics and communication skills exists across the range of clinical situations. It can be seen, for example, in considering informed consent; confidentiality; and in selecting couples for infertility treatment. And in many of these situations there are legal issues which any health professional needs to take into account.

The idea therefore behind the concept of practice skills is that good practice in medicine requires not only a knowledge of the scientific and technical aspects of medicine but also the necessary humanistic skills to put such knowledge into practice. These humanistic skills include:

(1) a sensitivity to the ethical aspects of a situation and an ability to think sensibly about them;
(2) an understanding of the legal framework within which the situation is set;
(3) an awareness of the patient's actual experience, and the experience of others involved (members of the health-care team as well as the patient's relatives), as the basis of the communication skills necessary to pull all this together in an effective treatment package.

The awareness of the patient's actual experience, which is certainly one part of the concept of patient-centred medicine, is therefore a component of practice skills. It is not surprising to find that patient-centred ideas have been helpful in many aspects of the project.

Details of the course and its scope are given elsewhere (Hope & Fulford 1994 a and b; Hope *et al.* 1995). In this chapter I will focus on the ways in which patient-centred ideas have been valuable in developing the course, and ways in which our experience in developing the course have helped to clarify the concept of patient-centred health care.

The meaning of patient-centred

Carl Rogers' concept of client-centred

The notion of patient-centred health care owes a great deal to Carl Rogers' concept of client-centred therapy (Rogers 1961). This notion was developed in the context of psychotherapy. Rogers later suggested using the broad term person-centred because the fundamental ideas had such apparently wide application (Rogers 1978). Rogers (1961) describes the characteristics of client-centred as:

> 'the therapist has been able to enter into an intensely personal and subjective relationship with the client – relating not as a scientist to an object of study, not as a physician expecting to diagnose and cure, but as a person to a person.... It would mean that the therapist is genuine, hiding behind no defensive facade, but meeting the client

with the feelings which organically he is experiencing ... and that he can convey something of his empathic understanding to the client.'

Elsewhere he summarizes the meaning of client-centred as 'meaning a person seeking help was not treated as a dependent patient but as a responsible client' (Rogers 1978).

Two aspects of the concept of patient-centred

It might be argued that medicine has always been 'patient-centred' because doctors traditionally do what is in the interests of their patients. Many doctors may feel angry at the suggestion that what they do is not patient-centred, because most doctors work very hard in the interests of their patients. If the criticism is that doctors focus on diagnosis and management, it may be countered that most patients' primary concern is for diagnosis and treatment. The key reason why the traditional medical perspective is not patient-centred is that it addresses what is for the good of the patient from the viewpoint of the doctor. Patient-centredness emphasizes the viewpoint of the patient. In the currently popular terminology of principles (Beauchamp & Childress 1994), patient-centredness is imbued more with the principle of autonomy, whereas traditional medicine values the principle of beneficence. But I do not believe that this formulation quite captures the essence of the concept of patient-centred medicine. At the root of patient-centredness is the valuing of the patient's perspective; it is not, as is the principle of autonomy, a principle to be used from a neutral, objective viewpoint. The principle of autonomy is putting a value on the patient's ability to control, but from the perspective of an objective standpoint. The patient-centred notion is subtly different: it is valuing the placing of the doctor in the patient's position. It is saying: see the patient from his own perspective. When you stand where the patient is, what do you see?

Although the traditional medical focus on diagnosis and treatment of disease does usually address the patient's primary concern, this focus is usually too exclusively on that primary concern. In other words, there are many things which are important to the patient, in addition to being cured, which medicine tends to underrate – to see as so trivial compared with the main job that it fails to address them at all. Several examples are given in Chapter 10 which describes the Planetree Experiment. One of the conclusions from this experiment is that it is important to pay attention to detail; for example, to the smell of the ward and to the quality of the soap.

Patient-centred ideas have been used by many people in the development of teaching, particularly of communication skills (Cohen-Cole 1991; Grant 1988; Pendleton *et al.* 1984). We have found these developments helpful in our own course. The part of our course which focuses on basic communication skills, for example, has been adapted from the approach developed by Pendleton and colleagues (1984), adapted because their approach was developed in general practice, whereas we are training medical students principally in the hospital setting. A number of tasks for the consultation are defined by Pendleton and his colleagues and these include:

- to define the reasons for the patient's attendance, including the patient's ideas, concerns and expectations;
- to choose with the patient an appropriate action for each problem;
- to achieve a shared understanding of the problems with the patient;
- to involve the patient in the management and encourage him to accept appropriate responsibility.

In adapting this approach to the hospital setting we have also made use of 'the three function approach' (Cohen-Cole 1991). The second of the three functions of the medical interview is 'developing rapport and responding to the patient's emotions'.

In the remainder of this chapter I will give some examples of the relationship between features of the Oxford Practice Skills Course and patient-centred ideas. In order to give the context for these examples I will first give a brief outline of the course as it has so far been developed.

Overview of the course

The main teaching consists of two principal strands:

(1) practice skills based seminars combining all three aspects of practice skills;
(2) small group tutorials which focus on basic communication skills.

The practice skills seminars are two hours long with an average number of 15 students. Each student takes part in three seminars in each of the three clinical years. The seminars have been enhanced by the use of both 'internal experts' (doctors and nurses working in the same clinical areas) and of 'external experts' (lawyers and philosophers). A summary of the core practice skills seminars is provided in Table 11.1.

The small group tutorials have been developed in collaboration between the practice skills project, the Department of Community Medicine and General Practice, and the medical tutor. Over 30 tutors have been trained (two-thirds are hospital doctors and one-third are GPs). Each group consists of five students and two tutors and meets ten times during the first clinical year for $1\frac{1}{2}$ hours each time. The topics of these tutorials are given in Table 11.2.

Patient-centred ideas and the practice skills course

Patient-centred ideas are relevant to all aspects of the course. I will consider these under three headings: syllabus, teaching methods, and evaluation and examination.

Table 11.1 The practice skills seminars. The course is spread across the three years of the clinical curriculum.

Title	Group*	Time	Setting
Year 1			
Introduction			
(1) An introduction to the practice skills course and tutorials in general communication skills	LG	2 hours	Introductory course
(2) Introduction to English and Welsh Law	LG	45 min	Introductory course
(3) Introduction to medical ethics	LG	45 min	Introductory course
Core practice skills seminars			
(4) 'Do not resuscitate'	SG	2 hours	General medicine
(5) Confidentiality	SG	2 hours	General medicine
(6) 'Have we got a consent form?'	SG	2 hours	General surgery
Year 2			
(7) Treating patients without their consent	SG	2 hours	Psychiatry
(8) 'We're desperate for a baby' (some ethical issues of assisted reproduction)	SG	1 hour	Obstetrics and gynaecology
(9) Anger and aggression in patients and their relatives	SG	2 hours	Accident services
(10) Consent to treatment and child abuse	SG	2 hours	Paediatrics
Year 3			
(11) Rationing health care: ethical issues	SG	2 hours	Medicine

* LG = Large group (100 students); SG = Small group (12–18 students)

Syllabus

Much of what is written in medical ethics concerns clinically rare situations chosen because they are philosophically interesting. One might call this philosophy-centred medical ethics. In choosing the syllabus of the practice skills project we specifically wished to address everyday medicine, and therefore to move away from philosophy-centred ethics. In moving away from philosophy-centred ethics we came to make a distinction between a doctor-centred and a patient-centred syllabus.

A doctor-centred syllabus focuses on dilemmas. A dilemma in this sense is a situation where a doctor becomes aware of an ethical problem raised by his or her practice. The key is that the doctor feels stuck

Table 11.2 General communication skills tutorials. All sessions take place during the first clinical year while students are attached to general medical and surgical wards.

Title	Group*	Time (hours)	Setting
(1) What is interviewing?	TG	$1\frac{1}{2}$	General medicine/surgery
(2) Structuring and use of time	TG	$1\frac{1}{2}$	General medicine/surgery
(3) Listening and questioning	TG	$1\frac{1}{2}$	General medicine/surgery
(4) Exploring patients' ideas, concerns and expectations	TG	$1\frac{1}{2}$	General medicine/surgery
(5) Explaining and sharing understanding	TG	$1\frac{1}{2}$	General medicine/surgery
(6) Introduction to breaking bad news	TG	$1\frac{1}{2}$	General medicine/surgery
(7) Breaking bad news	TG	$1\frac{1}{2}$	General medicine/surgery
Topics selected from:	TG	$1\frac{1}{2}$	General medicine/surgery
(8) (9) (10) angry patients; human sexuality; discussing outcomes – risk–benefit, going home – life after hospital; the garrulous/silent/tearful patient; patient taken overdose; working with colleagues/time economy			

TG = tutorial group (6–8 students)

and uncertain. I will give an example. In choosing the content of a seminar on confidentiality I gave the students a case vignette which posed a dilemma which they then discussed in small groups. The vignette concerned a man who was HIV positive but who did not want his wife to know. The issue was whether the doctor should breach confidentiality and tell the wife. Most doctors placed in this position would recognize that here is an ethical dilemma, even though many doctors may feel quite certain about what the right course of action should be.

At the end of the seminar a thoughtful student said that although the seminar was interesting it failed to address the most important aspect: the innumerable breaches in confidentiality which are routinely made by doctors and medical students. This feedback led me to rethink the seminar. Instead of thinking, 'what situations do doctors find ethically problematic in their day-to-day practice?' I asked instead, 'what situations and practices raise ethical issues which would be important to patients and which doctors do not notice?' The result has been that the first half of this seminar now consists of a discussion of breaches of confidentiality which occur and which health care staff rarely notice.

This represents a move, I believe, in the direction of a more patient-centred syllabus because it tries to address the question of what happens in medical practice that, from the patient's perspective, is unethical.

Teaching methods

In the practice skills course several teaching methods are used which give concrete realization to the idea of a patient-centred course. I will give several examples.

Role-play

We began using role-play as a method for students to practise their skills. The main focus of role-play was for the student to play the doctor. However, the value to students of playing the patient, or patient's relative, rapidly became apparent. Role-playing patients is a powerful way for students to understand patients' experiences. We have made increasing use of feedback from those students who play the role of patients. Indeed in some role-plays no one plays the doctor; for example, in one of the tutorials on breaking bad news (see Table 11.2) a video is shown. The first scene of the video is of a consultation of the patient with the GP. The patient has symptoms which are suggestive of cancer but some hospital-based investigations are required. The GP is honest and caring but does not address the woman's own worries.

After showing this scene, students are asked to role-play the woman returning home from the consultation and the ensuing conversation between her, her husband and her daughter. The purpose of this is for students to explore, through empathic identification with the woman and her family, the extent to which the consultation with the GP helped or hindered her and her husband in understanding and coping with her symptoms and worries. This role-play highlights the patient's need to be given an explanation and vocabulary which she can then share with the family. It is not obvious, until this role-play is carried out, that this is an important omission in the GP's consultation. Such understanding of the patient's situation cannot be achieved by passive observation, even if one is trying hard to see things from the patient's point of view.

Exercises

In larger seminar groups role-play can be problematic and cannot involve more than a few students. Exercises can be handled more easily in this setting and can be used to help students understand patients' perspectives. I will give two rather different examples.

In one of the early tutorials, when students are first learning on the wards how to clerk a patient and how to summarize the results of this clerking to the consultant, the following exercise is carried out. One student interviews another student for a few minutes about, for example, the experience of the first few weeks on the ward. The interviewer then summarizes this to a third student in front of the interviewee. Students who play the part of the interviewee frequently report feeling that their viewpoint has not been properly put across, and of finding it uncomfortable to be talked about in the third person over their heads. This exercise mimics the situation in which patients are 'presented' by junior staff to senior staff on bedside ward rounds.

The second example is taken from the core seminar on consent (Table 11.1). This seminar explores the idea of informed consent and its practical implications. One of the materials used is a video (Doyal 1991) showing a surgeon who is strongly (too strongly) recommending a mastectomy to a patient with breast cancer. The patient wants to have a lumpectomy. The surgeon wishes to maximize the chance of maximum survival. Later on in the seminar I present students with the following somewhat stylized situation: imagine that you have a disease for which there are two possible treatments. With the first treatment there is a 50% chance of cure (defined here as a healthy life for 50 years), and a 50% chance of death within a couple of days. The second treatment offers X years of healthy life. The question which I then ask students to decide, for themselves now, is this: what is the value of X that would make you unable to choose (be indifferent to) which of the two treatments to have. The original purpose of this exercise was to highlight the point that some people are risk takers and some are risk avoiders. The exercise is certainly a powerful way in which students realize the diversity of views amongst the group. In most student groups there is a wide range for the value of X from those who choose 5 years or less (one student chose 3 months) and those who choose 30 years or more. However, the main interest of the exercise lies in discussing what factors affect their choices.

For some, unless they are going to live long enough to complete their training, they feel they may as well risk almost instant death. For others the calculation is about having children and seeing those children to a certain stage in life. The student who chose 3 months argued that a 50% chance of death was a high risk and it would be a great pity to die without having had a really good time. He preferred a guaranteed few months in which to have 'a whale of a time' than to take that risk.

The exercise has a number of effects: firstly it forces students to consider a situation where they face a significant chance of a very much shortened life-span and where they have to make choices. This, I hope, gives them some insight into the situation which many of their patients face. Second, relating the exercise back to the video, it demonstrates that even amongst a group of people of similar age and background, there are fundamental differences in how they evaluate their life. I use this to emphasize how dangerous it is for the doctor to try and evaluate what 'is in the best interests of the patient' in the setting where the patient is faced with treatments with differing prognosis and differing effects. It has a third, and unpredicted, result which is important to the development of a patient-centred approach. It leads students to realize that we are all, potentially, patients. The concept of patient-centred health care forces a contrast between patients and professionals. At least for the purposes of teaching it is important for students to make use of the insight that they have been, and will be, patients.

Seminars off the wards

Although the intention is to keep the seminars close to the clinical work, the cases discussed are not normally current patients. This is in order to cover effectively a specific syllabus. Paradoxically this may help students to gain a more patient-centred view, because they can sit back from the immediacy of a situation, thus enabling them to imagine the situation from the patient's point of view. In the seminars students often say, 'if I were the patient I would want...'. Video material has a similar effect. The combination of its vividness and the fact that the student is not involved directly in the care of the patient portrayed, tends to lead students to identify with the patient's situation. The apprenticeship method of learning medicine, centred as it is around the care of actual patients, may strengthen students' identification with the medical profession and weaken their identification with patients. I am not suggesting that the apprenticeship model should be abandoned, but I think it is important that students also have the opportunity to stand back from actual practice.

Team teaching

One of the starting points in developing the practice skills project was that there should be team teaching – that several people should be involved in the teaching, including doctors and nurses who are working with the students on the wards. The original reason for this was to ensure both that the teaching becomes integrated with students' experience on the wards, and that students can learn the value of a team approach. A further effect of the team teaching has been that it provides a variety of perspectives on the issues under discussion. Nurses can often provide a perspective which is closer to patients' perspectives in some respects than is that of doctors. An unexpected effect of involving lawyers and philosophers in the seminars (which was done in order to enhance the academic content) is that they often speak from their experience as patients; they often provide a patient's perspective, unaffected by strong identification with the health professionals.

An obvious development, which a patient-centred approach suggests, is to involve patients themselves in the seminars and tutorials. This is an area of the teaching which we need to build up. Our experience so far highlights an interesting issue about a patient-centred orientation to teaching: who represents patients? In the context of individual patient care it is usually quite clear who the patient is, and it is therefore possible to identify the person who is at the 'centre' of patient-centred care. But in the context of teaching, where that teaching is addressing a generalized issue – consent or confidentiality, for example – who can represent the 'generalized patient'? We have found a wide diversity of views, for example, amongst patients who have taken part in the seminar on consent on the degree of involvement they would like in their own treatment.

Aspects of integration

Although I have argued that the seminars and tutorials can usefully offer students a setting in which they can stand back from the day-to-day work on the wards, it is part of the philosophy of the practice skills approach that the course is integrated into the rest of the clinical curriculum. There are a number of aspects of the course which are helpful in this:

(1) The teaching takes place throughout the three years; it is not carried out as a discrete 'full-time' course.
(2) The topics are related to the particular clinical work which the students are doing at that time.
(3) Doctors and nurses who are working with the students on the wards are invited to take part in the seminars (team teaching).
(4) The project office is positioned in a prominent place within the main hospital to which students have easy access.
(5) Those involved with the project take part in hospital and university activities and committees so that they play a part in the life of the hospital and medical school.

Integration is a two-way process: the teaching must fit with the clinical experience of the students; but it is also important that the students' clinical settings demonstrate patient-centred care. In the long run what may be more important is that the hospitals and other health care settings become more patient-centred.

Student-centred learning

The corollary of patient-centred health care is student-centred learning (Rogers 1961). However, it remains an empirical question (about which there is little good evidence) whether a student-centred approach to medical education helps to produce patient-centred doctors.

In the practice skills project we have involved students in a number of ways, although not specifically in order to promote patient-centred health care. Two students took part on the small working party which was set up at the start of the project to devise the structure of teaching and integrate it into the rest of the curriculum. Student feedback on the individual seminars has been collected, both formally and informally, and used to develop and improve the teaching. A part of each small group tutorial is a 'hot spot' which encourages students to raise issues which are of concern to them. Finally the topics for the last three of the small group tutorials (Table 11.2) are chosen by the whole group. There is room for further development of student-centred learning, and there may be good pedagogical reasons for developing in this direction; it remains uncertain, however, whether one reason is that it will promote a more patient-centred care.

Evaluation and examination

The evaluation of the teaching, and the examination of students in practice skills, are still at an early stage of development. We have used students' written responses to case vignettes as a basis for evaluating the course as a whole and are currently engaged in testing the reliability and validity of this method. However, since the teaching aims to improve actual practice, a better approach both for evaluating the teaching and for examining the students may be to devise situations using simulated patients – adopting the approach used in OSCEs (Objective Structured Clinical Examinations) (Hall-Turner 1983; Harden & Gleeson 1979) to the examination of practice skills. One of the advantages of this method, in keeping with a patient-centred perspective, is that it provides an opportunity for feedback on each student's performance from the (simulated) patient.

In the clinical examination, which students take at the end of their first medical and surgical attachments, examiners are recommended to ask students at least one patient-centred question, for example 'what is the patient's main concern?' or 'what is the patient expecting from this admission to hospital?'. By including these questions in students' first clinical examination we hope both to give the message that a patient-centred approach is important, and to ensure that students practise such an approach from the start of their clinical experience.

Conclusions

One important way of enhancing patient-centred health care is through the education of health profession students and practitioners. The Oxford Practice Skills Project represents a distinctive approach to the integration of ethics, communication skills and the law into clinical student education. In developing the course we have found the idea of patient-centred health care of considerable value, and our experience has helped our ideas of patient-centred care to develop.

Reading guide

A more detailed account of the Oxford Practice Skills Course is given in Hope and Fulford (1994) and Hope *at al.* (1995). Fulford's *Moral Theory and Medical Practice* (1989) argues in detail for the central role of values and the patient's experience of illness in medical concepts and practice. A briefer account is given in Fulford (1991). *The Journal of Medical Ethics* has an occasional section 'Teaching Medical Ethics'. Over the last ten years this journal has published many accounts of courses in medical ethics, particularly those in Britain but also some from other parts of Europe. The journal *Medical Education* publishes articles covering a range of relevant topics including methods of teaching and evaluation. A useful collection of articles on USA courses in ethics was published in *Academic Medicine* (1989) December, 64, 701–64. The teaching of communication skills to health professionals is addressed in Pendleton *et al.* (1984) which relates specifically to teaching general practitioners, and Burnard (1989) which is particularly useful for ideas for small group teaching. A good overview of Carl Rogers' ideas is to be found in the collection of his essays (Rogers 1961).

Burnard, P. (1989) *Teaching Interpersonal Skills: a Handbook of Experiential Learning for Health Professionals*. Chapman & Hall, London.
Fulford, K.W.M. (1991) The concept of disease. In: *Psychiatric Ethics* (eds S. Bloch & P. Chodoff), 2nd edn, pp. 77–99. Oxford University Press, Oxford.

References

Beauchamp, T.L. & Childress, J.F. (1994) *Principles of Biomedical Ethics*, 4th edn. Oxford University Press, New York.
Doyal, L. (1991) *The Nuffield Video Library in Medical Ethics and Law*. The Nuffield Foundation, London.
Fulford, K.W.M. (1989) *Moral Theory and Medical Practice*. Cambridge University Press, Cambridge.
Grant, V. (1988) Good communication vital for ethical practice. *IME Bulletin*, Nov., 13–17.
Grant, V.J. (1988) Doctor–patient communication: a five year training programme for medical students. *New Zealand Medical Journal*, **101**, 424–6.
Hall-Turner, W.J.A. (1983) An experimental assessment carried out in an undergraduate general practice teaching course (OSCE examination). *Medical Education*, **17**, 112–9.
Harden, R.M. & Gleeson, F.A. (1979) *Assessment of Medical Competence Using an Objective Standard Clinical Examination (OSCE)*. Association for the Study of Medical Education (ASME), Dundee.
Hope, T., Fulford, K.W.M. & Yates, A. (1995) *The Oxford Practice Skills Course Manual*. Oxford Practice Skills Project, Oxford.
Hope, T. & Fulford, K.W.M. (1994a) Medical education: patients, principles and practice skills. In: *Principles of Health Care Ethics* (ed. R. Gillon), Wiley, Chichester.
Hope, T. & Fulford, K.W.M. (1994b) The Oxford Practice Skills Project: teaching ethics, law and communication skills to clinical medical students. *Journal of Medical Ethics*, **20**(4), 229–34.
Pendleton, D., Schofield, T., Tate, P. & Havelock, P. (1984) *The Consultation: an Approach to Learning and Teaching*. Oxford University Press, Oxford.
Rogers, C. (1961) *On Becoming a Person*. Constable, London.
Rogers, C. (1978) *Carl Rogers on Personal Power*. Constable, London.

Commentary on Chapter 11

Donald McIntyre

In this chapter Hope offers a number of valuable insights on how ideas of patient-centred medicine have informed, or might further inform, his practice skills programme. I shall review these briefly and raise a few related questions.

It was helpful first to have a critical analysis of the term patient-centred and of its use. It is important to be reminded of how a term such as this, which describes something incontestably desirable, tends to be appropriated by a distinctive ideology and to be used as a political weapon to put others in the wrong. Hope properly starts his discussion with a reminder that most doctors and other health care workers see their work as patient-centred and are understandably angered by the aggressive use of the term by Rogers and his followers. Such anger, he points out, is justified in so far as 'most doctors work very hard in the interests of their patients and ... most patients' primary concern is for diagnosis and treatment'.

Nonetheless, at least in reflecting upon the practice skills course, he accepts the virtues of patient-centredness in the fuller ideological sense, and he emphasizes two aspects of this concept. Although '*most* patients' primary concern is for diagnosis and treatment', the patient-centred doctor is not content to base practice on that rule but commits herself to go the extra distance of finding out where the *individual* patient stands and of attempting to 'see the patient from his own perspective'. Secondly, although 'most patients' *primary* concern is for diagnosis and treatment', the patient-centred doctor is not content to limit her attention to the patient's primary concern, but also attends to other things which are of importance to the patient.

This highlighting of these two aspects of patient-centredness seems to me very helpful. On the one hand they make it clear that, other things being equal, this ideologically extended meaning of patient-centredness is also, like the basic idea, very difficult to contest as an ideal. On the other hand, this account of these two aspects leaves one in no doubt that each of them requires something extra from the doctor. To attend to the distinctive concerns of each individual, and to go beyond his priority concerns, is to add substantially to the work that the doctor has to do, to the time which she has to spend on each patient, and therefore to the costs of looking after each patient. If patient-centredness conceived in this way is an incontestable ideal other things being equal, it must also be noted that other things are never equal; for example, the extra resources which patient-centredness demands might conceivably be better spent, in the interests of patients' health, on rebuilding sewers, improved road safety or the alleviation of poverty.

The imaginative and carefully planned practice skills programme which Hope describes deserves to succeed and there can be no doubt that it will have a significant impact. However, experience suggests that complete success will depend on finding a solution to the endemic problem of the theory–practice gap. The importance of this problem stems from the fact that patient-centredness and other ideals embedded in the practice skills programme *are* ideals, both in the sense of being conceptions of what would happen in the best of all possible worlds and also in the sense of being abstractions which do not take account of all the specific practicalities of particular situations. It is likely that the experienced doctors and other health care workers encountered by medical students and junior doctors on the wards will, in their distinctive contexts and under the pressure of practical constraints, practise in ways which diverge significantly from these ideals; for example, where there is a tension between the time demands of patient-centredness and the need to diagnose and treat effectively the illnesses of all the patients in a crowded and understaffed ward, the ideal of patient-centredness is unlikely to be consistently maintained.

Furthermore, wherever there is a clear gap between the explicit messages novices receive from their professional education and the implicit messages they receive from the practice of experienced practitioners (and from what they themselves find possible in practice) it is almost inevitable that the messages from the educational context will in the end be dismissed as impractical theorizing. As Hope puts it, 'In the long run what may be more important (for professional education in practice skills) is that the hospitals and other health care settings become more patient-centred'.

That, however, may take a long time, and there are more immediate ways of dealing with the theory–practice gap implicit in another of Hope's comments: 'Although the intention was to keep the seminars close to the clinical work, the cases discussed are not normally current patients. This is in order to effectively cover a specific syllabus. Paradoxically this may help students to gain a more patient-centred view, because they can sit back from the immediacy of a situation thus enabling them to imagine the situation from the patient's point of view.' It is just such a clear distinction between the academic and clinical perspectives combined with the commitment to keep the two closely connected, which is central to any solution to the problem. There is, *pace* Hope, nothing paradoxical about the fact that it is in the academic setting that students can recognize the power and merits of patient-centredness and other ideals, and that different priorities will be uppermost for them in the clinical setting. What is needed is a clear and explicit recognition by all the staff involved, in both settings, and thence by the students themselves, that this kind of difference in perspectives is inevitable, that the different perspectives which are properly dominant in the two different kinds of setting are both important and indeed essential to good practice, and that the proper core of initial professional education is being introduced to the fruitful tension and the ongoing dialectic between these different perspectives. It is only in so far as students are clearly led, with the active support of their clinical teachers, to recognize the central importance of such a dialectic that one can expect the theoretical and idealized nature of their academic education to have a significant ongoing influence on their developing practice.

Finally, I want briefly to draw attention to the interesting connections and contrasts which Hope draws between patient-centredness and the other kinds of centredness. He points out helpfully the dangers of philosophy-centredness in that the problems which are most academically interesting may not be of great relevance to practitioners; but there is a need for some caution here. His concern to deal with issues that are practically significant is surely right, as is his concern to use cases and language which help to illuminate the practical significance of these issues; but it is an equal strength of his programme that it draws heavily on concepts and understandings of academic disciplines such as philosophy, the social sciences and legal studies: it offers academically powerful perspectives on practical issues.

Especially interesting is the relationship between student-centredness and patient-centredness which, as Hope points out, have been closely connected in Rogers' thinking. In the context of professional education for doctors and other health care workers, the tension between the two is worth noting; in any sense of the terms, student-centred and patient-centred agendas for professional education are likely to be quite different. Yet there are important similarities between the two ideas: for maximum effectiveness, professional education just like health care has to pay a great deal of attention to the distinctive concerns of the individual client, but on the other hand cannot allow uninformed or ill-judged client agendas to dominate expert judgement. In other words, in order to be useful, both have to be very sophisticated ideals.

12 ◆ A Case Study of a Patient-Centred Nurse

Angie Titchen

Nurses' stories sometimes reveal knowledge which is embedded in their clinical practice. This chapter is built around an interpretation of the actions and stories of an expert nurse who articulated her knowledge of patient-centred nursing, in particular how she used herself as a person in her relationships with patients.

Nearly 100 years ago, Florence Nightingale recognized that nursing is about taking care of the person who is ill, rather than attending primarily to medical problems. However, the hospital nursing service, developed in the west since Nightingale's time, has provided a service driven more by medical interests and nursing routines than by patients' experiences of their illness. Doctors were seen as knowing what is best for patients, with the nurse as 'doctor's handmaiden', supporting his or her work and helping patients to comply with doctor's orders. Patients were regarded as having little if any knowledge of their own bodies and as having little or no part to play in their own recovery. They were also seen as 'objects' to be cured and were depersonalized in hospital, for example by being referred to as 'the gall bladder in bed nine'.

Over the last 20 years, a new personalized style of hospital nursing has been developed which is driven by patients' experiences of their illness. The nursing profession uses the term patient-centred nursing to describe this style of practice – a style based on working with patients in partnership and on providing individualized, holistic care (attending to patients' particular psychological, social, emotional and spiritual needs as well as their physical needs). Patient-centred nursing is now being promoted in the UK. However, it is not widely practised and it is poorly understood.

My research is concerned with understanding what nurses who are expert in patient-centred nursing do well – from their perspective. I am using a phenomenological case study approach to investigate how they make sense of their professional craft knowledge or know-how – that part of their professional knowledge which they have acquired mainly through experience, in contrast to propositional knowledge of 'knowing that' which is derived through research or scholarship. Professional craft knowledge is a metaphorical term which I use to include all forms of nonpropositional knowledge; that is, practical, intuitive, experiential, aesthetic, personal and ethical knowledge (Higgs & Titchen in press). Such knowledge is usually tacit and embedded in practice (Benner 1984; Brown & McIntyre 1993; Polanyi 1958; Schon 1983).

Professional craft knowledge has both ontological and epistemological dimensions; that is, it is concerned, respectively, with our non-cognitive, spatial and temporal comportment or being-in-the-world, and with the often unconscious and unarticulated knowledge represented in our minds. These two dimensions make professional craft knowledge difficult to acquire through conventional teaching where knowledge has to be articulated. The purpose of my study is, therefore, to uncover the nature of professional craft knowledge of patient-centredness and to identify ways in which expert nurses can help less experienced nurses to develop this knowledge. The significance of the work overall is the drawing out and making use of such knowledge to improve the quality of patient care. In this chapter I present the nature of the professional craft knowledge of Alison Binnie, a senior sister and expert in patient-centred nursing, in a busy acute medical ward at the Oxford Radcliffe Hospital. The ways in which she helped other nurses to learn are not explored here.

To capture both the epistemological and ontological dimensions of professional craft knowledge, I devised a methodology which uses ideas from two distinctive, but complementary, phenomenological traditions. Schutz's (1967, 1970) phenomenological sociology has an epistemological concern and is a rigorous approach to the study of the obvious, through bringing the phenomenon as fully to consciousness as possible. Heidegger's (1962) hermeneutic phenomenology has an ontological concern and is the laying out of something that is not already obvious. That something is the sense and ground of the obvious and must be made to show itself. My research strategy, based on observing, listening and questioning (Titchen & Higgs in press), was designed to bring the phenomenon of patient-centred nursing as fully to consciousness as possible and to lay out its sense and ground. The research methods were participant observation, indepth interviews and review of documentation (including Alison Binnie's and staff nurses' unpublished papers). Data were analysed using a rigorous and systematic approach (Titchen & McIntyre 1993) to generate contextualized, interpretive, abstract accounts of nurses' professional craft knowledge. All names, except Alison's, have been changed to protect the identity of the participants.

In this case study, I draw particularly upon Campbell's (1984) Christian theological interpretation of professional care because Alison claimed that his imagery and concepts helped her to clarify and make sense of what she did, from a secular perspective. My grounding of Campbell's concepts in empirical data provided by an expert nurse, offers something new because Campbell primarily uses biblical stories and Christian doctrine to illustrate his concepts. Where he uses empirical findings, they are limited to studies of traditional nursing practice to illustrate possibly undesirable opposites of the concepts, rather than the concepts themselves, for example 'doing to' as opposed to 'being with'. This work has, therefore, gone further than Campbell's, by uncovering knowledge about how a nurse can be, and work as, a skilled companion.

'Taking yourself as a person into the relationship': skilled companionship

> *Alison Binnie (AB) (Written paper)* 'For me, the essence of patient-centred nursing has become developing a relationship which enables me to address my patient's personal experience of health or illness. Then, within this relationship, I offer a special companionship and a range of practical skills which, together, if the patient is willing to accept them, have the power to transform his experience.'

Alison believed that helping people who are ill happens through a relationship and that 'the relationship between the individual nurse and the individual patient is absolutely central' to the delivery of care. Every relationship between nurse and patient is unique and within it both the nurse and the patient are valued as people. Nurses use themselves as the main instrument of nursing to engage with the patient as a whole person. They use their intellect, bodies, emotions, sensitivity, interpersonal skills.

> *AB: (Written paper)* 'Being effective, being therapeutic as a nurse means, for me, helping a patient to move from an unsatisfactory or problematic position to a more positive and healthy one. It means accompanying and assisting a person in the transition from illness to wellness, from pain to comfort, or from distress to coping. Campbell's (1984) notion of the nurse as a skilled companion who accompanies a person on a journey until he is ready to go his own way, has been helpful and influential here. Campbell describes this companionship as a 'delicately balanced relationship' in which the nurse's sensitive presence, her willingness to recognize the nature of the patient's very personal journey and share in it, is as important as the practical or technical skill she may use to smooth his path.'

Binnie considered that nursing is often a journey with a patient into the unknown and is, therefore, risky. She also believed that 'taking yourself as a person into the relationship' and working effectively with the whole person, required a well developed self-knowledge and maturity.

To dispel the outdated ideas of the nurse as 'doctor's handmaiden' or 'ministering angel', Campbell (1984) created fresh imagery for dedicated caring by describing nursing as 'skilled companionship'. He chose the concept to describe a relationship which is 'professional without being distanced or manipulative' and a physical closeness that is not sexually-oriented. The concept also implies movement and change.

My interpretation is that the kind of relationship that Alison described implies a partnership between the nurse and patient. Partnership suggests an egalitarian relationship which does not currently exist, partly because of socialization and partly because of the vulnerability of the person who is ill. To undo decades of socialization into acceptance of depersonalized patients, I suggest that Alison revealed the essential features of her knowledge of persons, that is, particularity and mutuality. She articulated her knowledge of 'particularity', a concept used by Campbell to mean moving from one's generalized knowledge to the individual case, so that care is tailored specifically to the individual person. Particularity requires 'mutuality', Campbell's concept to describe 'being with' patients, rather than just 'doing to'. 'Being with' or, in Alison's words, 'working with', means that nurses have to understand their patients' inner world of experience if they are to help them. Exploration of her knowledge using these concepts will take us on to her knowledge of how she expressed her care through the use of her body, using Campbell's concept of 'gracefulness'.

'Who is this person and where are they?': particularity

Alison saw each patient as different and special and needing to be nursed accordingly. Providing care that was 'individually tailored to the patient's needs' means that patients had to be carefully assessed.

> *AB: (Written paper)* 'For me, assessing a new patient is an infinitely variable interpersonal process, not a predetermined procedure. The process is adapted according to the patient's condition and how he responds to me, and according to other demands within the ward. But in some way or other, I spend time being with the patient and, at some stage, his family too. I listen to his story, as he presents it, encouraging or empathizing in whatever way seems helpful at the time. I try to discover "where he is at" and what his perceptions and concerns are. As I listen, my nursing observational skills are at work, partly at a conscious, partly intuitive level. I pick up cues that my professional knowledge enables me to recognize as significant and worthy of further exploration. As the conversation proceeds, or maybe at a later stage, I ask questions that arise from the patient's story or from what I have observed or sensed. In this way I begin to get to know the patient and his family and build a relationship with them.'

The patient's own story formed the agenda in the assessment. Alison explained that if the nurse has a heavy agenda, she may give listening a lower priority than the questions that she feels are imperative to ask. Alison explained why it was important to discover 'where the patient is'.

> *AB: (Written paper)* 'I cannot join my patient on his journey unless I know where he is starting from. Discovering my patient's starting point, or to put it colloquially, understanding "where he is", means addressing his *experience* of his current situation ... The work of Benner and Wrubel (1989) has helped me greatly in appreciating, as a nurse, the value of addressing a patient's ... lived experience of health and illness as the major focus of nursing work...'

The *Tim and the Orange* story below, shows how she uses her knowledge of 'where the patient is' to help the patient to move on.

Tim and the Orange

AB: (Interview) 'The patient had been in hospital feeling unwell and with rather vague symptoms, profuse sweating, fevers, vomiting, diarrhoea and had had a whole battery of tests that had not produced any answers. Not surprisingly he was getting rather low in spirits... At 11 AM one morning, a nurse asked me if I would go and spend some time with him, because she didn't know what to do with him; he didn't want to get out of bed. I remember going into his room and finding him lying dishevelled, unshaven, hot and sweaty in a very crumpled bed. He looked lethargic and miserable. I sat on his bed with him for a few minutes, not saying very much at all, just with my hand on his hand. I could feel inside me quite a strong desire to get him out of bed, get him in the bath, washed and get his bed freshened up and I knew if we could do all that, he would feel better. I also knew that if I suggested such a line of activity he would resist strongly because it wasn't at all what he was feeling like. So I just sat and waited for some initiative to come from him.

After a period of silence, he said, "Do you know what I have been dreaming about? I've been dreaming about a fresh orange; I want to suck on a fresh orange"... So I got an orange from the kitchen and brought it back, peeled and nicely presented, cut up into small segments. He said he thought that he was allergic to oranges and it would probably make him sick, but it was what he wanted more than anything else. I thought that it wouldn't matter too much if it did make him a bit sick if he ... felt, or could recognize that I was trying to respond to his needs, as he saw them.

So I sat on the bed with him as he sucked away on his orange. He told me that he hadn't eaten anything for four days and that he thought it had something to do with why he was feeling so weak and lethargic. There were very few things that he fancied to eat and very few things that didn't make him feel sick or have diarrhoea. While I listened to him and we talked together gently, he did come up with a few suggestions of things he might be able to tolerate ... Limited though they were, we did manage to find out a number of things he could cope with....

Having started at a point where he was at, wanting an orange, I gently built up some trust and confidence with him and felt able to tentatively suggest that he might like to have a bath. He said that he felt that he couldn't cope, that he wouldn't have the energy; so I suggested taking him in a wheelchair and sitting him on a seat in the shower. He said that he would try that. So I did exactly that ... really freshened him up, helped him to shave, change, gave him fresh sheets... He was very weak and he did find it very tiring, but he really felt better afterwards, he felt much more positive and was very pleased to have made the effort.

This little story represents, for me, two important things in nursing practice. First, it is about starting work with patients wherever they are at; not rushing in and imposing what you want to do right at the start. But if you can start where they are at, you can help them to move in a positive direction. You can work therapeutically in that way. The other thing this illustrates is the detailed work of individualized nursing. It illustrates the fact that I believe it is attending to these minute details – a desire at that moment for a fresh orange – allowing a person to express these personal whims, desires, accepting them and being able to meet them in helpful ways, that often makes a great difference to how a patient feels.'

One interpretation of this story is that Alison was valuing, and building on, Tim's knowledge of his own body, so that she could attend to the particularity of his needs. She was aware that in order to respond creatively, rather than predictably, she needed information from her patient about what would help restore his strength at his own pace. I suggest that she was adopting a phenomenological approach to nursing (Benner & Wrubel 1989; Harvey 1993) because she was seeking out her patient's perspective and building on it to help him to feel better. She knew that merely imposing her own knowledge of what would help would be unsuccessful.

Another interpretation concerns the time and attention demanded of professionals when they use knowledge about illness and health which is based on generalizations and return to the individual case. Alison attended to and made time for this return in a busy ward, by prioritizing and 'focusing down in detail on certain things'. This return requires moving away from sameness and predictability and seeking the new and different (Campbell 1984). Alison sought out the unorthodox in her everyday work with Tim. By responding to his desire for a fresh orange at that moment, she was able to develop an understanding of his unique world and to work out with him a few things that he could eat. This work shows the close connection between particularity and mutuality.

Alison believed that it was important to convey the uniqueness of the patient as a person to other members of the team:

> *AB: (Written paper)* 'I want nurses reading my assessment to be confronted at once with a human being who has a history and a place in society ... I select the relationships, events and experiences that seem to have been most significant in shaping the course of the person's life and the person he or she became ... key facts about the patient's life will help others to relate to him as an individual, to see him in the context of his social position and background and as part of a social network ... These key things will help others to relate sensitively to the patient as they build their own relationships with him.'

Nurses using Alison's care plans said that their first reading gave them a 'whole picture of the patient', 'I feel as though I have met the person'. Her patients felt that they had been 'treated as a whole person' and that she really understood their problems and needs. Some particularly noted her acceptance of their spiritual needs, whilst recognizing that she did not necessarily share their beliefs.

In summary, Alison demonstrated the concept of particularity through her awareness that her professional knowledge alone is insufficient to help other people towards wellbeing and a realization of their hopes and aspirations. She recognized that she must be able to understand others' worlds from their perspective and that this means relying on 'the revelation of an inner world of experience, to which there is no access from the outside, except so far as the other person chooses to grant it' (Campbell 1984).

'Working with': mutuality

Alison's belief that nurses should work in partnership with their patients was put into practice in a number of ways. She tried to work creatively with the patient, and sometimes with relatives as well. In her view, the *Tim and the Orange* story captures the essence of how she works with her patients, by responding to their needs as they see them, rather than imposing on them what she felt was best. In this story, I suggest that Alison was recognizing that particularity required mutuality 'with the aim of improving knowledge' (Campbell 1984). Offering acceptable help to the patient required a meeting of the world of the patient and the world of the expert nurse.

If professionals take mutuality into account, Campbell (1984, p. 107) proposes that 'we feel cared for when our need is recognized and when the help which is offered does not overwhelm us, but gently restores our strength at a pace which allows us to feel part of the movement to recovery. Conversely, a care which imposes itself on us, forcing a conformity to someone else's ideas of what we need, merely makes us feel more helpless and vulnerable'. The special knowledge of the nurse can, therefore, be used as a form of domination, if the nurse imposes what she thinks is best for the patient. We get a sense that Tim experienced a restoration of strength because help was designed and paced with knowledge which he offered, suggesting that Alison avoided such domination by 'curbing her strong desire' to get him out of bed and to freshen him up.

When writing a nursing care plan, Alison tried to avoid using jargon, so that her patient would feel involved in the care planning process. She considered that jargon could be alienating for patients and she tried to make her language understandable, without being patronizing. One of her patients, Neil, and his wife, Rebecca, described the experience of sharing of care planning:

> *Rebecca:* (*Interview*) 'sharing care and what was really happening, what their hopes and fears were, what the treatment was, all this was outstanding – very open and helpful.'
> *Neil:* 'They used laymen's language...'
> *Rebecca:* 'I would read the charts and the care notes and I was encouraged to do so. It wasn't saying, "what are you doing looking at that?", (rather), "the notes are there, read them if you wish".'

Another way that Alison worked with patients was by including them and their relatives, if present, in professional discussion at the bedside. Alison frequently looked at the patient for confirmation, as she told another nurse what had been happening that day. Eye contact and the expression on her face said, 'Have I got this right?'. Devices were used to give the patient a voice in the discussion:

> *AB:* (*Interview*) 'You start a sentence talking to the nurse ... and you say, "He's not been feeling very well today", and then you complete the sentence

talking to the patient saying, "Have you?" So that's actually a grammatically incorrect sentence, but it works to switch halfway.'

Other devices included asking the patient to tell the nurse coming on duty what had been happening that morning or what the results of tests were. I suggest that these devices enabled Alison to share responsibility with patients for handing on accurate information and to give patients opportunities to present their own views, interpretations or needs.

Working with patients also included collaboration with families. Traditionally, families are not included in the care of their relatives and are often asked to leave if some procedure is to be carried out. The following stories show how Alison involved relatives in physical forms of caring – if they wanted to.

I might easily have pushed her out of the way

AB: (*Interview*) 'A sick lady had just had an amputation and I had found her early in the morning to be in severe pain. I gave her a strong analgesic injection and made her comfortable and left her. That was a carefully planned decision, knowing that she would probably be able to sleep for a while and then I'd be able to move her without causing too much pain... Later, as I was working with another patient behind the screen, I heard her daughter arrive and say, "Oh, you haven't had a wash yet; you've still got your hospital gown on" – slightly critical remarks. I had been planning to go to this lady next and bath her. So there was this slight feeling of the daughter criticizing everything when I'd planned it so carefully! But I was totally aware of that and went out and greeted the daughter and got her to help me. I had heard her get out things and fill up a bowl; she was going to wash her. So I joined in and got the daughter to help me and gave her a clear role in it ... I didn't want her to feel put out. You know, you can see how in the traditional role, you might easily have pushed her out of the way ... I went in and explained in a very gentle voice – not critical of her – what I'd done that morning and why ... I had to do it for my own sake, but it was important that the daughter didn't feel I had left her mother all morning. It turned into a very nice activity – she did everything with me, apart from change the sheet.'

In this story, Alison appears to be accepting the daughter's wish to be involved in her mother's care. The following account shows another dimension, that of explicitly giving permission to relatives.

Fieldnotes: 'Miss Cox, a former nurse, had been nursing her mother at home for some years and now, as her mother was dying, she wanted to continue to look after her in the ward. She said that Alison allowed her to do this and that her contributions and suggestions were welcomed and taken up. "This is the only place where I haven't had a fight to be involved in the care of my mother."'

In relation to the concept of mutuality, I theorize that Alison recognized that her relationships with patients and relatives were not naturally egalitarian ones because patients are vulnerable and dependent to varying extents on the nurse. To work with patients and relatives in facilitative relationships, rather than 'doing to' or imposing what she believes is best for the patient, she saw that she had to equalize power within her relationships. By not using jargon, Alison demystified professional care and facilitated patients' and their families' contribution to care planning. Her behaviour gave patients and relatives permission to be involved in care, and consequently they felt that they had a legitimate contribution to make. These actions allowed patients and relatives to share responsibility with her and to enter into more equal relationships. She helped them to move from a position where the nurse is seen to know what is best, to one where knowledge of what is best proceeds from a meeting of the helper and helped (Campbell 1984). This movement was achieved by adopting the role of facilitator which involved a personal risk of being sometimes shown to be imperfect. Only by taking such risks can a nurse truly enter into facilitative relationships.

'Using the body': graceful care

Using her body to communicate care, Alison tried to convey to patients, 'I am here for you' by being unhurried and gentle in her movements and by being physically close and touching them when she was talking with them. She usually sat on the bed or chair, or kneeled or crouched on the floor, with a hand on the patient's hand, arm or shoulder. Her eyes were either level or below those of the patient and eye contact was sustained. Her face was often only about nine inches away from the patient's. This closeness was deliberate; she was trying to create a private space for her patient talk without others being able to overhear their conversation. She always listened intently and was rarely distracted. She gave time for patients to respond, sometimes allowing long silences with sustained eye contact and a gentle, encouraging expression.

The story of *Tim and the Orange* illustrates, I suggest, how Alison used her body: 'I sat on his bed with him for a few minutes, not saying very much at all, just with my hand on his hand ... I just sat and waited for some initiative to come from him.' Her physical closeness penetrated the haze when Neil was very ill. He was confused and paranoid and thought that 'all the nurses and doctors were actually there to do me harm ... it was a sort of delirium'.

> *AB: (Interview)* 'Neil said that, in the haze, he kept seeing my face and he came to feel that it was safe and he said, "I decided in my confusion to make a commitment to Alison".'

Two staff nurses observed Alison help Robert, an elderly gentleman, to have a wash in bed:

> *JH and HF: (Written paper)* 'Alison took the opportunity, given by the wash, to let him talk about his life. There was no discussion about the wash itself, it flowed smoothly and became incidental to their conversation. The total attention she gave him allowed her to quickly tune in to him.'

Later Alison reflected upon this interaction:

> *JH and HF: (Written paper)* 'What I feel is important, is a total focus on the patient... That's quite difficult sometimes with the distractions and you're busy ... except it becomes part of a way of practising ... I think that is quite powerful for the patient, the patient senses this total attention. Although other things are going on in my mind sometimes, there's still this part of me that really just attends to the patient and that is very accepting and listening, quite still if you like. I try to put over a kind of stillness.'

Campbell (1984) suggests that 'the experience of being cared for, rather than being "managed", is summed up in the adjective 'graceful'. He argues that gracefulness in caring is closely associated to bodily expression. Physical care given by nurses to bedridden patients is genuinely caring if it is gracefully administered, that is, 'carried out in a way that is appropriately sensuous, with a tender respect for the disabled person'. In all Alison's stories we catch a glimpse of her comportment through her use of body in time and space. We see her bodily expression of attunement, tenderness and acceptance, through her stillness; a stillness created by her smooth, unhurried and gentle movements, gentle voice and facial expression and sustained eye contact. Thus she affirmed her focus on patients' and relatives' concerns and her genuine openness and receptivity to their experience. This bodily expression created a feeling of safety and trust and comforted, supported, nurtured and reached out to frightened, depressed and withdrawn patients.

Conclusions

I have suggested that Alison articulated her knowledge of 'taking herself as a person into the relationship', through Campbell's (1984) analogy of the 'skilled companion' accompanying the person on his/her own very personal journey. I have extended the analogy to describe, analytically, interpretively and contextually, the know-how embedded in her practice and in her being, as a nurse and person. Essential features of her knowledge of people – the concepts of particularity and mutuality – could be discerned in her stories. So, too, we have been able to distinguish one area of her knowledge of self in the concept of graceful care. These concepts are embodied in the development and sustaining of facilitative relationships with patients and their families. Relationships are established by equalizing power and through asking the question, 'who is this person and where are they?' to access the patient's unique world and knowledge. Thus the nurse creates the opportunity for working with patients and families and the part patients play in their own care is legitimized As well as uncovering this epistemological dimension of knowledge, the essential ontological dimension has been revealed. The way nurses *are* in the world – the way they comport themselves – is also an essential part of *being* a patient-centred nurse.

Reading guide

Patient-centred nursing

There are no empirical or theoretical works which specifically investigate the nature of patient-centred nursing as a style of nursing. This is astonishing in today's climate where patient-centred nursing is seen to be the aspiration of both the nursing profession and the government. Reference to patient-centred nursing is to be found in the literature relating to primary nursing (when a philosophy of patient-centred nursing is espoused), therapeutic nursing and the study of expert nurses. Literature on nurse–patient relationships is also relevant.

Binnie, A. & Titchen, A. (in press) *Patient-centred Nursing in Practice: a Study of the Development of Primary Nursing in an Acute Medical Unit.* National Institute for Nursing, Oxford.

Macleod, M. (1990) *Experience in everyday nursing practice: a study of 'experienced' ward sisters.* Unpublished doctoral thesis. University of Edinburgh, Edinburgh.

McMahon, R. & Pearson, A. (eds) (1991) *Nursing as Therapy.* Chapman & Hall, London.

May, C. (1992) Individual care? Power and subjectivity in therapeutic relationships. *Sociology,* **26**(4), 589–602.

Morse, J.M. (1991) Negotiating commitment and involvement in the nurse–patient relationship. *Journal of Advanced Nursing,* **16**(4), 455–68.

Pearson, A. (1988) *Primary nursing – nursing in the Burford and Oxford Nursing Development Units.* Croom Helm, London.

Phenomenological approach to nursing

Paterson, J.G. & Zderad, L.T. (1988) *Humanistic Nursing.* National League for Nursing, New York.

Tanner, C.A., Benner, P., Chesla, C. & Gordon, D.R. (1993) The phenomenology of knowing the patient. *IMAGE: Journal of Nursing Scholarship,* **25**(4), 273–80.

Taylor, B.J. (1992) From helper to human: a reconceptualization of the nurse as a person. *Journal of Advanced Nursing,* **17**, 1042–9.

Phenomenological views of the person in nursing research

Benner, P. (1985) Quality of life: a phenomenological perspective on explanation, prediction, and understanding in nursing science. *Advances in Nursing Science,* **8**(1), 1–14.

Leonard, V.W. (1989) A Heideggerian phenomenologic perspective on the concept of the person. *Advances in Nursing Science,* **11**(4), 40–55.

Professional craft knowledge

Agan, R.D. (1987) Intuitive knowing as a dimension of Nursing. *Advances in Nursing Science,* **10**, 63–70.

Carper, B.A. (1978) Fundamental patterns of knowing. *Advances in Nursing Science,* **1**(1), 13–23.

Lawler, J. (1991) *Behind the Screens: Nursing, Somology, and the Problem of the Body.* Churchill Livingstone, London.

Manley, K. (1991) Knowledge for nursing practice. In: *Nursing: a Knowledge Base for Practice* (eds A. Perry & M. Jolley), pp. 1–27. Edward Arnold, London.

McCormack, B. (1992) Intuition: concept analysis and application to curriculum development. 1. Concept analysis. *Journal of Clinical Nursing,* **1**, 339–44.

Reason, P. & Heron, J. (1986) Research with people: the paradigm of co-operative experiential enquiry. *Person-Centred Review,* **1**, 457–76.

References

Benner, P. (1984) *From Novice to Expert: Excellence and Power in Clinical Nursing Practice.* Addison-Wesley, London.

Benner, P. & Wrubel, J. (1989) *The Primacy of Caring: Stress and Coping in Health and Illness.* Addison-Wesley, Wokingham.

Brown, S. & McIntyre, D. (1993) *Making Sense of Teaching.* Open University Press, Buckingham.

Campbell, A.V. (1984) *Moderated Love.* SPCK, London.

Harvey, S. (1993) The genesis of a phenomenological approach to advanced nursing practice. *Journal of Advanced Nursing,* **18**, 526–30.

Heidegger, M. (1962) *Being and Time.* Harper & Row, New York.

Higgs, J. & Titchen, A. (in press) Propositional, professional and personal knowledge in clinical reasoning. In: *Clinical Reasoning Skills* (eds J. Higgs & M. Jones). Butterworth Heinemann, Oxford.

Polanyi, M. (1958) *Personal Knowledge.* University of Chicago Press, Chicago.

Schon, D.A. (1983) *The Reflective Practitioner: how Professionals Think in Action.* Temple Smith, London.

Schutz, A. (1967) *The Phenomenology of the Social World.* Northwestern University Press, Evanston.

Schutz, A. (1970) *On Phenomenology and Social Relations* (ed. H.R. Wagner). University of Chicago Press, London.

Titchen, A. & Higgs, J. (in press) Facilitating the use and generation of knowledge in clinical reasoning. In: *Clinical Reasoning Skills* (eds J. Higgs & M. Jones). Butterworth Heinemann, Oxford.

Titchen, A. & McIntyre, D. (1993) A phenomenological approach to qualitative data analysis in nursing research. In: *Changing Nursing Practice Through Action Research* (ed. A. Titchen). Report No. 6, pp. 29–48. National Institute for Nursing, Oxford.

Commentary on Chapter 12

Peter Jarvis

There are four crucial issues in Titchen's chapter to which I wish to respond: the issue of patient-centred nursing; the idea of the expert; personhood; practical knowledge. Finally, brief note is included about the nature of professional preparation in the light of the chapter to which I am reacting.

Patient-centred care

Throughout the chapter runs the theme of patient-centred care which I want to question, but not in order to return to nurse-centred care! The idea of patient-centred care conjures up pictures of nurses acting on patients, doing things for them, almost as if patients are impersonal 'its'. Nurse-centred and patient-centred are treated as if they are the only alternatives; they reflect the individualizing nature of contemporary society which encourages this assumption. Indeed, it is an element in the 'risk society' criticized by Beck (1992) in his assessment of modernity, since individuals are removed from support relationships. I want to introduce a third idea – relationship-based nursing. There is confusion between this and patient-centred care since exponents of the latter often refer to the significance of relationships, and this certainly occurs in Titchen's chapter.

Buber (1959) raised a significant point when he suggested that in the beginning is relationship, and all 'real living is meeting' (1959). Buber's work is less frequently studied these days than perhaps it ought to be, but Levinas (1989) returns to it and raises significant points about it which are important here. He writes:

> 'The presence of the other, ipso facto, implies a 'word' which is addressed directly to me and which requires a response. Whoever refuses to reply, no longer perceives the "word". It is impossible to remain a spectator of the Thou, for the very existence of the Thou depends on the "word" it addresses to me. And it must be added, only a being who is responsible for another being can enter into dialogue...'

Levinas continues that only through meeting can there be dialogue in which both truth and commitment can be experienced. Only in relationship is it possible for the moral values of humanity to appear, so that we need to return to these fundamentals in professional practice and in so doing break away from the problematic moral values implicit in the individualization that has occurred in this modern age.

However, it should be noted that patient-centred care is itself a reaction to another prevalent form of modernist behaviour – proceduralism. We live in an impersonal bureaucratic world which functions to ensure that social interaction is smooth and unemotional. But human beings are not like that, as Titchen notes. Her expert nurse regards nursing as embarking upon a risky journey into the unknown – human relationships are always like this. The risk is tremendous, but if it is successful then the outcome is good. There are risks in entering relationships, including the fact that we are expected to perform specified procedures, and failure to do that might appear unprofessional.

However, there is another. If the patients themselves reject the relationship because they expect proceduralism, then this can be even more problematic. Procedures and proceduralism can inhibit the development of relationship-based care, which can be frustrating if they are expected to perform specified duties, but it can be even more frustrating if nurses find that the patients judge them by their ability to perform the procedures rather than by their capacity to create a caring relationship in which healing and growth can occur.

The expert

This is no criticism of Alison Binnie, whose work appears to fit much of what I believe to be central to nursing, but it is important to define 'expert' with great care, and this is rarely done. Expertise is a modern concept; it suggests technical skill and sophisticated knowledge. These are important in nursing, but they are not enough. Levinas (1989) suggests that theories of knowledge are also theories of truth. Now, truth can only be discovered in relationship, so that the truth of the patient can only be discovered in relationship-based nursing. Indeed, Binnie is recorded as saying that she cannot join her patient 'on his journey unless I know where he is starting from'. The point about this is that the nurse can have the most sophisticated knowledge and can perform all the nursing procedures with tremendous skill – but if she cannot build relationships she cannot gain sufficient knowledge of the patient to become a nurse of the type whom Titchen describes as expert.

The idea of personhood

The idea of personhood follows from this and demands little comment here, although Levinas' (1989) summary of Buber perhaps epitomizes the position adopted here:

> 'The I–Thou relation is a relation of true knowledge because it preserves the integrity of the otherness of the Thou instead of relegating the Thou to the anonymity of the It.'

Only through relationship can personhood develop and those who live with procedures and impersonality are inhibited in their human development. Human being is always becoming in relationship, and this is an essential element in caring.

Practical knowledge

Nursing is about people and practice; epistemology and ontology are related. That relationship, however, needs discussion. Nevertheless, practical knowledge – Titchen calls this professional craft knowledge – starts from both knowledge of the person and theoretical knowledge of nursing (see Jarvis 1991 for a discussion of the concept of theory). These two forms of knowledge come together in practice and constitute the basis of practical knowledge. But practice is risky, as Alison Binnie pointed out, and this must always be the case if the journey with the patient is into the unknown; herein lies the basis of practical knowledge – pragmatism. Heller (1984), writing of everyday knowledge, points out that pragmatism denotes the unity of theory and practice, since the expert acts with sufficient ground to produce the best possible results, and she is always adjusting her behaviour in response to the person with whom she is relating.

Titchen suggests that the expert nurse found it easy to articulate her practical knowledge, but what she seemed able to do was to talk about relationships and there are few incidents in which she describes the precise nursing skills being used. Perhaps this is because practical knowledge is harder to articulate and was lost in the discussion about personal relationships. Practical knowledge, argues Nyiri (1988), is 'tacit, non-propositional and ... inarticulable'. He goes on:

> 'One becomes an expert not simply by absorbing explicit knowledge of the type found in textbooks, but through experience, that is, through repeated trials, "failing, succeeding, wasting time and effort ... getting a feel for a problem, learning to go by the book and when to break the rules". Human experts thereby gradually absorb "a repertory of working rules of thumb, or "heuristics", that, combined with practical knowledge, make them expert practitioners. This practical, heuristic knowledge, as attempts to simulate it on a machine have shown, is hardest to get at because experts – or anyone else – rarely have the self-awareness to recognize what it is. So it has to be mined out of their heads painstakingly, one jewel at a time".'
> (All quotes from Feigenbaum & McCorduck 1984)

Conclusions

Nurses, then, have to be trained as people who work in and through relationship, a neglected area of nurse education. This is both professional and personal education, but it must be central to the preparation for nurses who work in relationships with their patients, and this form of professional preparation needs to be carefully developed. There is always a danger that this approach to experiential education of denigrating professional knowledge in order to incorporate the personal and apparently practical. But good practical knowledge must also be theoretical. Consequently, it is no good tinkering with professional education in order to appear to produce nurses who relate to patients; it is necessary to reconsider the nature of professional education itself. The educator of nurses is more than just one who transmits nursing knowledge to new recruits; he/she is the guardian of a tradition about the meaning of nursing into which new nurses are inducted. It is fitting, therefore, that this commentary should end where it began – with Buber (1961) who wrote that 'Education worthy of the name is essentially education of character', and the character of the nurse is as important as the knowledge that she possesses.

References

Beck, U. (1992) *Risk Society*, trans. M. Ritter. Sage, London.

Buber, M. (1959) *I and Thou*, 2nd edn., trans. R.G. Smith. T&T Clark, Edinburgh.

Buber, M. (1961) *Between Man and Man*, Fontana edn., trans. R.G. Smith. Collins, London.

Feigenbaum, E. & McCorduck, P. (1984) *The Fifth Generation*. Signet, New York.

Heller, A. (1984) *Everyday Knowledge*, trans. G.L. Campbell. Routledge, Kegan and Paul, London.

Jarvis, P. (1991) Practical knowledge and theoretical analyses in adult and continuing education. In: *Erwachsenenbildung im Kontext* (eds M. Friedenthal-Hasse, J. Reischmann, H. Tietgens & N. Vogel). Klinkhardt, Bad Heilbrunn.

Levinas, E. (1989) Martin Buber and the theory of knowledge. Reprinted in *The Levinas Reader* (ed. S. Hand). Blackwell Publishers, Oxford.

Nyiri, J. (1988) Tradition and practical knowledge. In: *Practical Knowledge* (eds J. Nyiri & B. Smith). Croom Helm, London.

13 ◆ Needs, Rights and the Duty of Care Towards Patients of Radically Different Cultures

Len Doyal

In recent years, a moral and legal consensus has evolved about the rights of patients. Two moral principles are more or less presupposed by professional codes, an ocean of academic commentary and much common law. The first states that clinicians should use their expertise to protect life and health to an acceptable professional standard. The second proclaims that they should respect the autonomy of their patients – their right to self-determination. In a clinical setting, this latter duty translates into subsidiary principles of informed consent, truth telling and confidentiality.

Elsewhere I have developed a meta-ethical justification of a strongly deontological interpretation of the duties of clinical care, as well as analysed the degree to which most clinical encounters fail to conform to a rigid interpretation of these duties (Doyal 1990, 1994). In this chapter, I will apply some of these arguments to the practice of medicine in a multi-ethnic community where patients and their clinicians may not share the same moral values. Such cultural differences raise three questions which I will address.

First, can the preceding duties of care really be said to be universal or are clinicians guilty of cultural imperialism when they adhere to them? Second, if we accept the universality of these duties, how can we improve their application to clinical encounters with patients from very different cultural backgrounds? And third, what is the most morally appropriate action when there is a direct clash between accepted duties of care and competing cultural values?

Universal and objective human needs

In our book, *A Theory of Human Need*, Ian Gough and I argue that it is possible to identify universal and objective human needs (Doyal & Gough 1991). Briefly, the structure of our argument is:

(1) All humans in all cultures have an objective interest in participating in some form of life due to links between the development of individual potential and social interaction.
(2) In order to avoid disabled participation – serious harm – individuals must satisfy the basic needs of survival/physical health and autonomy. The latter entails the presence of sufficient under-

standing, emotional confidence and social opportunity for successful social participation to be a meaningful possibility.

(3) The degree of serious harm – of disabled social participation – will vary inversely with the degree of need satisfaction. The chance of successful social participation will increase with the degree to which individuals possess physical health and autonomy.

(4) 'Intermediate needs' specify the universal satisfier characteristics required for the successful satisfaction of the basic needs for physical health and autonomy (e.g. adequate nutrition, appropriate health care, education, and physical and economic security). While intermediate needs are universal, their adequate satisfaction can take a variety of cultural forms. Human needs can therefore be seen to be universal without this culturally dictating how individual needs should be satisfied.

(5) What we call 'critical autonomy' entails the capacity not just to act creatively within a culture but also to be able to reject the values of that culture in favour of another. Individuals can be highly autonomous within a culture but still, conceptually, emotionally and practically, imprisoned within it.

The right to optimal need satisfaction

We further argue that everyone, everywhere has a right to optimal levels of need satisfaction. To argue that an individual has a right to something is to make a very serious claim. It is to maintain that an entitlement exists which others have a strict duty to respect.

Some writers have suggested that needs in themselves entail the existence of welfare rights (Goodin 1988). We reject this view. The existence of the right to basic need satisfaction follows instead from the belief that others have moral duties on which they should act – whatever the cultural values concerned. Different forms of social life implicitly or explicitly share a common vision of the good. The good person is the individual who does her or his duty, as prescribed by the values of the culture or subculture of which they are a part.

The imposition of duties of moral goodness logically entails at least two things on the part of those who impose them (Gewirth 1978; Plant *et al.* 1980). First, they must believe that those on whom these duties are imposed have the right to basic need satisfaction in the terms already outlined. Diminished physical health and autonomy disable social participation. Due to such disablement, potentially good persons will not necessarily be able to do what is expected of them. The imposition of duties of moral virtue, however this might be culturally construed, without the right to basic need satisfaction is therefore contradictory.

Thus what does it mean for me to expect you to be a morally good person in my terms? Presumably there are a range of things which I want you both to do and to refrain from doing; acts of both commission and of omission. Yet for you to do either, you must possess appropriate levels of physical health and autonomy in the preceding terms. Acts of commission associated with physically active social interaction – e.g. engaging in professional activity to a designated moral standard – will usually demand high levels of both types of need satisfaction. Even acts of omission requiring no ostensible physical action – e.g. your doing nothing to interfere with my chosen activities – entail minimal levels of physical health along with the cognitive capacity to understand the social meaning of the omission, and the emotional capacity to act accordingly (Plant 1992).

Second, if the imposition of strict moral duties on others entails the right to basic need satisfaction, the question remains of how much satisfaction is required for it to be met. The simple answer is as much as is available for moral agents to do their best. Suppose, for example, that those who impose visions of *their* good expect less than the best of those on whom the visions are imposed. This might be through not providing them with access to the intermediate need satisfiers and the consequent levels of physical health and autonomy which they require in order for them to do their best. This would be inconsistent with the moral commitment of those imposing their values on others. They could not believe that their good was that good after all! If you take your moral values seriously – whatever their cultural content – then you must wish for me to do the same and as well as I can.

Taking rights seriously and the clinical duties of care

The right to optimal need satisfaction has been shown to carry with it corresponding duties. Translated into a clinical environment, these turn out generally to be the professional duties of care with which we began: to protect the life, health and autonomy of patients to an acceptable standard. These arguments are based on reason and not moral intuition. From the perspective of their own moral commitments, all clinicians believe that both they and their patients have certain duties. One of these is to be a good patient: once patients have chosen to have medical treatment, they should act responsibly through doing their best to follow whatever plan of medical management has been prescribed.

For such beliefs about the moral responsibilities of patients to be consistent – for patients to be able to do their best to comply with the medical advice which they are given – their basic needs must be satisfied. They must have the physical, intellectual and emotional competence to act accordingly. This in turn implies that clinicians must strive to do what they can to optimize this competence. Such a derivation of the primary duties of care places a distinctly deontological interpretation on how principles of beneficence, nonmaleficence and respect for autonomy should translate into clinical practice. Deliberate deception is not acceptable, for example. For as a result of the deceit, the patient would not be able actually to do the very things which probably prompted the deceit in the first place – to take charge of their life (or what is left of it) in a way that conforms to the clinician's own vision of the good.

The problem of moral indeterminacy

The complexity of individual clinical consultations sometimes imposes what I have called a 'moral indeterminacy' on the duties of care (Doyal 1990). For example, at the beginning of diagnosis and treatment it may be reasonably obvious what it means to protect the physical health and to respect the autonomy of a newly diagnosed diabetic. However, where does one stop in the face of continued refusal to follow medical advice?

Autonomy is not like a single attribute which individuals either do or do not possess. It should rather be regarded as a spectrum of intellectual, physical and emotional skills which vary in relation to the social opportunity for them to be learned. This is why patients who do not possess high levels of autonomy pose such a moral problem when they appear to be making decisions which go against a wide consensus of professional opinion. The middle class diabetic who gives perfectly cogent reasons why he or she does not wish to live under the constraints which medical compliance would impose may be clinically frustrating. However, there is nothing indeterminate about our duty of care toward them. If it is clear that they understand the consequences of their actions, we let them get on with it and bring up their compliance again when , say, their condition deteriorates to the point that they may wish to review their choice.

Yet if the patient appears to be ignorant of the nature and hazards of their condition, uninterested in learning, inarticulate, angry and non-clinically depressed, their decision is hardly as autonomous as the first. This is the case, irrespective of the fact that the decision is still autonomous in that it is their choice, even though we may not be quite sure what the choice is.

Most clinicians specialising in diabetes would rightly regard it as inappropriate simply to accede to the noncompliance of the competent patient with low levels of autonomy. Rather clinicians will typically counsel, educate, cajole and in other ways pressure the patient to understand why their actions are self-destructive and what they can practically do about it – if they so choose.

Thus far we have focused on the problems of moral clarity posed by patients with low levels of autonomy in relation to their clinical care. Of course the same can be said of the autonomy of their clinicians who may well lack the intellectual and emotional abilities to follow through in moral practice what they know they should attempt in principle (Davis & Fallowfield 1991).

It follows that the determinacy of moral decision making in medicine will be based in part on a consensus of what good medicine ideally entails and the possession by patients and clinicians of the requisite levels of autonomy required to approximate it in practice. Yet until medical education dramatically improves, clinicians will continue to lack autonomy in a variety of ways. As regards patients, the scope for improvement is even more vast, incorporating every aspect of the provision of social welfare in a rapidly deteriorating welfare state.

Thus there will always be some moral dilemmas posed by clinical cases where it is still unclear how best to proceed. Here, the most that can be expected is for the decision making process to be as rational as possible. This will entail the curtailment, for example, of vested interests but most important, a prominent and coherent voice for patients or their representatives.

Of course, we must always err on the side of caution. The right of competent patients to act as the gate keepers of their own bodies must be respected, even if the levels of autonomy which they display as regards their care are low and they may not understand the full implications of their actions. Yet we must also recognize that to say that clinicians or patients *ought* to act in specific ways presupposes that they can. To abstract moral principles from the practical preconditions for their implementation is little more than an exercise in self-indulgence.

Taking the rights of patients seriously in circumstances of radical cultural difference

What follows from the preceding analysis about the rights of patients of 'radical cultural difference'? For our purposes, this will mean people whose primary pattern of beliefs, moral values and language are fundamentally different from those of the clinicians who treat them. However, to polarize cultures in this way poses serious anthropological problems, especially in the context of Britain where there is a great deal of normative overlap between different beliefs and values within the population (Archer 1988).

The group on which I shall focus – the Bangladeshi community in the East End of London – is hugely varied in its relation to the wider culture. While for some there is a significant convergence of values with the wider culture, for others there are profound cultural and linguistic differences (Currer 1986). Their systems of belief are focused on the Islamic faith, on fate as a key determinant of life and death events, on a strict division of male and female labour, on the crucial importance of honour in making moral decisions and on a very strong sense of duty to conform to traditional values. Against the background of what for many is poverty, social standing is closely related to cultural conformity which is often enforced with intense fervour. In treating patients of such radically different culture, the universality of the two duties of care continues to dictate that clinical provision is directed toward the satisfaction of objective basic need. Let us examine the practical implications of each duty in turn.

First, the obligation remains to provide clinical care to a high standard. The Bangladeshi community has rich traditions of folk and lay healing to which members experiencing illness will often turn as a first resort (Helman 1990; Kleinman 1986). When this fails, therefore, patients who present for orthodox treatment are often in great physical need. For by this time, their participation within their community may have been seriously compromised by disease and their personal experience of it.

The care on offer is 'western' in that it is derived from the concepts, techniques and methodologies within the biomedical model. I have argued elsewhere that the diseases and associated disabilities which lead patients of whatever cultural background to seek such care will best be dealt with through the competent employment of this model (Doyal 1987). Obviously, clinicians who use it must take care not to confuse the beliefs and activities of patients which are alien to them with ignorance or psychological abnormality (Qureshi 1989). For obvious reasons, such confusion can affect the potential success of treatment, limiting the willingness of distressed and angry patients to comply with medical advice. It can also lead to misdiagnosis (Fernando 1991).

The second universal duty of care dictates that the autonomy of all patients should be respected, whatever their culture. What this means in principle is clear. If, through withholding information, clinicians subject patients to therapeutic procedures which they clearly do not understand when consent to them is obtained, then their autonomy and their rights are being abused. As regards the autonomy of patients of radically different culture, there are many examples in practice of what such abuse entails. In the case of Bangladeshi women who are about to give birth, for instance, it is important to try always to organize obstetric resources so that men will not be present, or to obtain the woman's consent if this is difficult. Another example is for clinicians to use available translation services and to provide explanatory literature in the language of the patient. More often than not, access to both is lacking because of inadequate resources. This should mean the clinician spending as much time and effort as possible to achieve optimal levels of understanding (Putsch 1985). In principle, cultural diversity should not interfere with clinical respect for autonomy.

Back to the problem of moral indeterminacy

We have argued that the universality of human rights demands equal respect for all, irrespective of culture. Yet as we have already seen, what is clear in principle can be opaque in practice. This can be especially dramatic with patients of radical cultural difference. On the one hand, how should one proceed clinically if the need is great but the level of understanding for informed consent is poor? On the other hand, at what point should one clinician stop attempting to respect the apparent 'autonomy' of patients who are clearly not making choices for themselves? Both questions are part of the daily moral texture of clinical work at the interface of extreme differences of culture and language. Sometimes there are no clear solutions.

As an example, consider a Bangladeshi woman who speaks poor English, has a long history of heart disease and now requires urgent surgery for an aortic aneurism. She has consistently posed moral problems for her cardiologist because her husband insists on accompanying her and on answering all questions put to her. The diagnosis and treatment of her disease has required clear communication. Yet it has seemed strange to her that she should be in charge of communicating important information about herself – even information of this personal kind. As a result, she has been reticent to participate in the consultation except through the medium of her husband.

The moral indeterminacy of this situation is clear. In the circumstances described, some clinicians will just do the best they can to obtain an accurate history, believing that clinical information should only be obtained on the patient's own terms. If this agreement is culturally mediated in ways which are less than clinically optimal, then so be it. Yet doubt will remain about the patient's real wishes and about the morality of possibly compromising her clinical interests as a result. Communication about pain, for instance, has been shown to be culturally influenced (Wolff & Langley 1977). Misunderstanding about cardiological symptoms can obviously take place as a result. Proceeding in the way described will mean that the error, if there is one, will be on the side of respect for what is hoped to be the patient's autonomous choice to let others speak for her.

But the same moral drama can be played in reverse. Here clinicians may become so frustrated by their inability to communicate with the patient or to dissuade the husband from interfering in the process, that the latter will be asked to leave. The justification might be in relation to protecting the patient's health or respecting her autonomy without the interference of others. If this demands restricting the consultation so that her usual deference to her husband does not interfere, then so be it. If patients choose to refuse to co-operate in the provision of effective care then there is no clinical duty to provide it ineffectively.

Things get even more complicated when we move to the aneurism itself. This is a risky procedure and ordinarily there would be no question but that considerable attention would be paid to obtaining informed consent before proceeding. Yet under the circumstances, it is the very importance and drama of the choice to be made that can make the wife even less willing to attempt to discuss the matter without her husband present. Indeed, in such circumstances, it may strike some patients as bizarre that they have an individual decision to make at all (Sen 1990). For aside from her perception of her husband's authority, important decisions are very much focused on the family. Therefore the patient may appear surprisingly detached about her fate, especially in the light of her often further belief in its predetermination (Currer 1986).

Suppose this woman's agreement to the surgery takes the form of immediately accepting her husband's instruction to sign the consent form. Should the surgeon proceed without insisting that more time is spent discussing the situation with the woman and the translator alone? How much time? Again, one can argue the case either way. Where the condition is seriously and immediately life threatening, there is little doubt that intervention should proceed provided that agreement – as opposed to informed consent – has been obtained. Yet this would hardly be regarded as acceptable when dealing with patients with similar cultural beliefs.

What should be done in these circumstances is to continue to search for ways of improving the ability of clinicians to communicate across cultural boundaries and to educate patients of radically different culture about the principles which clinicians are professionally and morally obligated to employ in their treatment. As regards clinicians, this will mean more attention throughout medical education not just to medical ethics and communication skills but also to medical anthropology. The more clinicians understand about why intellectual and emotional barriers exist to biomedicine, the better able they will be to negotiate them successfully with their patients. Of equal importance is a drive to recruit more medical students from radically different cultural backgrounds.

For patients, better translation facilities are crucial as are translations of existing educational material about health and health care. Literature should not just be in the primary language of patients but should attempt to describe typical problems in encountering biomedicine in the cultural terms of patients themselves. At the same time, steps should be taken to try to make the environment of clinical care – for example changes in decor, dress or background music – less culturally alienating than it so often is at present. The more it is possible to create a more acceptable transition between home and the institution of care, the more clinicians who are able and willing can in practice respect the autonomy of patients of radical cultural difference – without compromising their clinical care (Helman 1990).

One important experiment which has put some of these ideas into practice involves 'health advocates' from the same ethnic background as patients of radical cultural difference. Trained to represent the rights of patients against the background of an intimate understanding of their cultural values, these new health professionals are available to better inform patients about health and clinical matters and to liaise between patients and clinicians when problems of ethics or communication are identified. This can involve the resolution of conflict between patients and clinicians or between patients and their families. Through giving patients better information and trying to ensure that they have an effective voice in the clinical decision making process, advocates can influence both the content and the outcome of clinical practice (Parsons & Day 1992).

These proposals represent one strategy of improving the ability of clinicians to respect the rights of their patients of radically different culture. The implementation of such proposals will not solve the problem of moral indeterminacy but will minimize it as much as is practically possible. At the same time, it is important that morally complex cases are discussed by as many members of the health team as possible. Different individuals will have varying moral perspectives, professional experience and anthropological and linguistic skills relevant to the problem at hand, and the most rational course of action will be the one which has been most effectively debated. The fact that with hindsight a decision may appear to have been the 'wrong' moral choice only underlines the importance of everyone concerned knowing that it was made with an acceptable degree of collective deliberation.

Where culture, morality and reason collide

Thus far our discussion of cultural conflict has been consistent with the theory of rights and clinical duties developed earlier. Even in circumstances of cultural conflict where the choices of patients might be at odds with those of their clinicians, the moral importance of autonomy dictates respect for their choice. Where it is unclear how to conform to these ideals in practice, clinicians are still not brought into direct conflict with the patient's radically different culture because of their respect for the patient's autonomy. For however difficult it may be for patients to understand clinical information and to communicate their related choices, they rightly will not expect their choices to be ignored, whatever their cultural orientation.

Yet anomalies remain which can lead to even more dramatic clashes between cultural values than the ones outlined thus far. For example, it has already been noted that the idea of the individual as the moral focus of important decision making is inconceivable in the context of some radically different cultures. Take the principle of confidentiality as an example. Provided that the patient agrees to open ended communication with relatives, then of course there is no moral problem. However, when there is disagreement – for example, an 18 year old daughter who has had an abortion or a 38 year old wife who has had a sterilization, both of whom wish for their privacy to be respected – there can often be major conflict.

The father or husband may demand clinical information in the confidence that many if not all of the members of his immediate community support his belief in his entitlement to it. He will be especially insistent if he believes that the information might have serious implications for the future of his family. In short, within some radically different cultures, there is no strict right of confidentiality and thus little respect for autonomy. From his perspective, he might not be able to fulfil his primary social role as family head – that of protector of its honour – without this information (Kabeer 1990).

Yet the right of the daughter and her mother to have their autonomy respected should trump the cultural imperatives of the father. We have seen that his belief that he should be able to insist that they do as he wishes is contradictory – even as regards his own moral expectations. He cannot expect the daughter or wife to be able morally to conform to his vision of the good without respecting the autonomy which they require to do so. Cultural conformity can always be bought at the price of slavery. Enforced conformity should not be confused with the conformity of adherence to moral duty which has been chosen on the basis of an understanding of alternative possibilities.

In such circumstances, clinicians can be thrown into direct conflict with radically different cultural norms. We have seen that respecting the ordinary autonomy of patients means respecting choices which are understood to be an expression of the culture of which they are a part. However the duty of care extends to respect for critical autonomy and may well entail supporting patients in their rejection of some of the values of their primary culture, usually because they perceive its representatives as ignoring their individual interests in some fundamental way.

Thus at times the duty of care demands actions which by implication are culturally discriminatory in the face of values which do not take human rights seriously. Again, to force anyone to adhere to a vision of your good – rather than respecting their right to the basic need satisfaction required to make an informed choice that it is the good – is morally wrong for everyone, everywhere. Respect for critical autonomy can even lead to clinicians being justified in resisting – though not ultimately ignoring – the immediate choices of patients. In these circumstances there is a tension between respecting a short term expression of autonomy within cultural boundaries, and respecting the need for critical autonomy – the development of the capacity to choose between such boundaries.

Smokers of whatever culture may rightly be told – even when they make it clear that they do not want to listen – that if they do not stop, they may deprive themselves of making any choices in the future. The same can be said of many cultural conflicts in a clinical setting. At worst, they may simply reflect ethnic prejudice on the part of the clinician. At best, such conflict can reflect a commendable attempt to help patients to understand that short term decisions which may seem warranted by their cultural values may be inconsistent with promoting their long-term health. For example, a woman may urgently need to control her fertility to maintain her physical health, but for cultural reasons may find this difficult to accept or even discuss. One way of respecting her autonomy is to accept her decision to reject sterilization or even contraception without further comment. Yet we know from previous experience that she may alter her choice after counselling. How to balance respect for autonomy in the short-term with respect for critical autonomy in the longer term is morally indeterminate for the reasons we have seen. What is clear is that the decision to focus on the latter will constitute an implicit rejection of the cultural values on the basis of which her initial choice is made (Moore 1988).

Finally, and at the extreme, clinicians should not agree to participate in cultural practices which because of associated physical damage also severely limit the critical autonomy of their victims (James 1994). The moral horror of female circumcision, for example, is not just the terrible circumstances in which it is sometimes inflicted on young girls. Clinicians could correct these. The horror points to the future – of health risks associated with reproduction and of the foreclosure on a range of physical and psychological experiences and choices which will be denied the child involved (Lightfoot Klein 1989). Of course, similar arguments can be applied to clinical work within the dominant culture which would result in limiting the critical autonomy of patients, even if they are desired in the short term (e.g. some forms of plastic surgery).

None of this should be surprising. To the degree that we accept the universality of human rights and understand the duties of clinical care as following from such rights, conflict will be inevitable if the cultural beliefs of patients and their families do neither. While such conflict is not common in clinical practice within a multi-ethnic community, it will occur in work with patients of radical cultural difference. When it happens, it is crucial to ensure that it is not based on misunderstandings. In these circumstances collective discussion among the health care team will again be important and will need to include advocates with a background in the cultures of the patients involved. Of course, in the face of whatever moral indeterminacy remains, all that can be asked is that clinicians do the best they can to respect the basic needs of their patients.

Conclusions

In this chapter I have argued that the clinical duties to protect health and respect autonomy can be derived from my theory of human need and rights developed with Ian Gough. I then showed how what might be morally clear in principle often becomes indeterminate in practice, depending on the levels of physical health and autonomy of patients and the educational and communication skills of clinicians. We saw how this same indeterminacy can dramatically increase when medicine is practised in multi-ethnic communities with dramatic cultural contrasts, and we explored approaches to minimizing its consequences. Finally, where it proves impossible to respect both the rights of patients and particular types of cultural belief, it is the latter which must be sacrificed. The universality of the basic human rights from which the duties of care derive demands no less.

Acknowledgements
Many thanks to Rosemary McKechnie, Sheila Hillier, Alistair McDonald, Sabiha Choudry and especially Lesley Doyal for their help and advice.

References

Archer, M. (1988) *Culture and Agency*, p. 19. Cambridge University Press, Cambridge.

Currer, C. (1986) Concepts of mental well- and ill-being: the case of Pathan mothers in Britain. In: *Concepts of Health, Illness and Disease* (C. Currer & M. Stacey), pp. 181–98. Berg, Leamington Spa.

Davis, H. & Fallowfield, L. (1991) *Counselling and Communication in Health Care*, pp. 3–58. Wiley, London.

Doyal, L. (1987) Health, underdevelopment and traditional medicine. *Holistic Medicine*, **2**(1), 27–40.

Doyal, L. (1990) Medical ethics and moral indeterminacy. *Journal of Law and Society*, **17**(1), 1–16.

Doyal, L. (1994) Needs, rights and the moral duties of clinicians. In: *Principles of Health Care Ethics* (ed. R. Gillon), pp. 217–30. Wiley, London.

Doyal, L. & Gough, I. (1991) *A Theory of Human Need*. Macmillan, London.

Faden, R. & Beauchamp, T. (1986) *A History and Theory of Informed Consent*. Oxford University Press, New York.

Fernando, S. (1991) *Mental Health, Race and Culture*, pp. 113–45. Macmillan, London.

Gewirth, A. (1978) *Reason and Morality*. University of Chicago Press, Chicago.

Goodin, R. (1988) *Reasons for Welfare*, pp. 27–50. Princeton University Press, Princeton.

Helman, C. (1990) *Culture, Health and Illness*. Wright, London.

James, S. (1994) Reconciling international human rights and cultural relativism: the case of female circumcision. *Bioethics*, **8**(1), 1–26.

Kabeer, N. (1990) Poverty, purdah and women's survival strategies in rural Bangladesh. In: *The Food Question: Profits versus People* (eds H. Bernstein, B. Crow, M. Mackintosh & Martin), pp. 135–48. Earthscan, London.

Kleinman, A. (1986) Concepts and a model for the comparison of medical systems as social systems. In: *Concepts of Health, Illness and Disease.* (C. Currer & M. Stacey), pp. 27–50. Berg, Leamington Spa.

Lightfoot Klein, H. (1989) *Prisoners of Ritual: An Odyssey into Female Genital Circumcision in Africa*. Haworth Press, New York.

Moore, H. (1988) *Feminism and Anthropology*, pp. 12–41. Polity Press, Oxford.

Parsons, L. & Day, S. (1992) Improving obstetric outcomes in ethnic minorities: an evaluation of health advocacy in Hackney. *Journal of Public Health Medicine*, **14**(2).

Plant, R. (1992) Citizenship and rights. In: *Liberalism, Citizenship and Autonomy* (eds D. Milligan & W.W. Miller), pp. 108–33. Avebury, Aldershot.

Plant, R., Lesser, H. & Taylor-Gooby, P. (1980) *Political Philosophy and Social Welfare*, ch. 3–5. Routledge, London.

Putsch, R. (1985) Cross-cultural communication. *Journal of the American Medical Association*, **254**(23), 3344–8.

Qureshi, B. (1989) *Transcultural Medicine*. Kluwer, Dordrecht.

Sen, A. (1990) Gender and co-operative conflicts. In: *Women and World Development* (ed. I. Tinkler), pp. 123–49. Oxford University Press, New York.

Wolff, B. & Langley, S. (1977) Cultural factors and the responses to pain. In: *Culture, Disease and Healing: Studies in Medical Anthropology* (ed. D. Landy), pp. 313–19. Macmillan, New York.

Commentary on Chapter 13

Roger Crisp

Let me begin by saying how much I agree with many of the conclusions Doyal reaches in his stimulating chapter. In particular, I am sure that he is right to suggest that clinicians should protect the health of patients within the bounds set by patients' autonomous and informed decisions. I agree also with this thesis of 'moral indeterminacy', as well as his final suggestion that when morality and cultural beliefs conflict there is no reason to respect the beliefs instead of morality. One might even make out an argument that this is analytic – that is, that it follows from the fact that the reasons we are looking for here are themselves moral. In practice, of course, even in a case of conflict between morality and cultural beliefs, any conflict will consist in a difference of belief. The conflict is to be resolved in favour of one set of beliefs only if those beliefs are correct. So there is room here for some caution on the part of clinicians.

Unlike patient-centred care, the ideal of which revolves around a relationship of mutual agreement, philosophy advances, if at all, by disagreement. So in the rest of my brief response I want to note my three main areas of disagreement with Doyal.

Logic

Doyal claims that any clinician who believes that patients have certain moral duties, such as to act responsibly, is logically committed to the view that patients have a right to the satisfaction of their needs. Imagine a hard-nosed libertarian doctor who denies that there is any 'positive' right to anything whatsoever, but who says that patients in hospital should act responsibly. Doyal's argument that this doctor is committing a logical fallacy rests on the assumption that this doctor believes that it ought to be the case that patients are acting responsibly. For patients to do this, their needs must indeed be satisfied. But the doctor may not believe this. Rather she may believe that *if* patients find themselves in hospital, then they ought to act responsibly. If people die, perhaps because they have no money and their needs cannot therefore be satisfied, that is bad luck for them. But they have no right to the satisfaction of their needs. This is an unreasonable view, but it is not illogical.

Needs

Doyal's argument invokes the notion of need. I agree that the question of what people need, and how best to satisfy their needs, is important both in philosophical theory and in clinical and political practice. But an argument grounded on needs does not go deep enough, since an unsatisfied need provides no reason to act. The following example should illustrate what I mean.

The HIV virus needs certain conditions if it is going to survive: basically, that plenty of people engage in unprotected sex and use dirty needles. But the fact that the virus needs these conditions does not provide anybody with any reason – even a weak, overridable reason – to do these things.

Surely, however, we do want to say that people's basic needs to health care should be met? Yes, but not because they are needs. The reason to provide health care is grounded on what people need it *for* – that is, a good life. In other words, the satisfaction of basic needs in the case of human beings is instrumental to something good in itself which is independent of basic needs.

The instrumentality of needs actually emerges in Doyal's discussion. He talks, for example, of the avoidance of 'harm'. This does indeed provide part of the basis for the justification of a health care system. But because he concentrates on the notion of need, the conception of human wellbeing underlying his account remains undeveloped. He stresses the value of social participation. But there is more to a good life than this. Consider for example the values of understanding the world, pleasure, and personal accomplishment. This concentration on social participation also makes it harder to defend autonomy. According to Doyal, autonomy is a need which must be met if a person is going to engage in worthwhile social participation. But consider Ms B. Let us imagine that she is quite incapable of the exercise of autonomy in that she always defers to her husband on any significant question. We can nevertheless still suggest that her personal relationships enable her to flourish. A more plausible account would go beyond need to wellbeing itself. One component of wellbeing is the exercise of autonomy. The harm this woman suffers is the deprivation of autonomy itself, not the damage to her capacity for social participation.

Rights

In the previous section I started by saying that the notion of need is important in medical ethics, even if there are other more important notions lying behind it. In this section, I want to make a stronger claim about the notion of rights: we can do without it. Consider the following case, again adapted from the same example in Doyals' chapter.

A doctor is investigating Ms B., who requires urgent surgery. When she defers to her husband, the doctor throws the husband out. He then threatens Ms B. into signing a consent form, and she is admitted to surgery immediately. I hope that everyone will agree that this doctor had a strong reason not to do what he did. This reason is primarily that he violated the autonomy of the patient. But notice that we can say that the doctor had a strong reason to respect the patient's autonomy without any talk of rights, or indeed of duties.

So what? you might say. Why is it important which moral concepts we use? The answer is, clarity. Our moral language contains concepts from a host of past traditions and we should not be unreflective about the concepts we have been left, since they may involve confusions or be unnecessary. In other words, each concept we employ must earn its keep. The concept of rights cannot do this, and can be eliminated without loss. More positively, eschewing talk of rights will prevent our spending time in developing a logic of rights which may result in actual distortion of our moral critical faculties. Just as needs are *for* certain goods or the absence of bads, so the rights people speak of are *to* certain goods or the absence of bads. It is these that provide our reasons for action, and it is conceptions of these that should provide the focus for our discussions in medical ethics.

V ◆ *Audit and Feedback*

14 ◆ Patient-Centred Health Care and Complaints

Linda Mulcahy with Sally M.A. Lloyd-Bostock

The whole notion of patient-centred care may be confusing to those who believe that provision of all health care services should be patient oriented, the goals being to diagnose, cure, relieve and counsel. The fact that the term patient-centred has been coined at all suggests that these goals are not being met and that the efforts of those in the health service need to be refocused. This stance is one which has been adopted by the consumer lobby over recent decades and which has prompted much debate about how the ideal is to be achieved.

The phrase patient-centred begs many questions. Does it involve total empowerment of the patient through the expression of needs and preferences? Is there a role for the professional or the state in the assessment of need or shaping of preferences? To what extent are claims to a patient-centred approach in competition with other claims? Does patient-centred care take account of the collective needs of patients or just those of individual patients? What happens when collective and individual needs are in conflict?

In this chapter we consider some of these issues with reference to one of the 'services' provided by hospitals in England: the procedure for making and responding to complaints. We outline the NHS hospital complaints procedure and discuss the various perspectives from which one could judge whether the complaints procedure is patient-centred. We address three main issues. First, do complaints systems meet the standards required of any state mandated system for redress of citizen grievances? Second, viewed from an organizational perspective do they satisfy the collective needs of the patient population by using complaints to improve the quality of services? Third, seen from a complainant perspective, do they satisfy the needs of individual complainants?

The relationship between patient- and complainant-centred approaches

The term patient-centred is not necessarily a suitable one to use in the context of complaints systems since not all complaints are made by, or involve, patients. Evaluations of service may be made by relatives, carers, friends, pressure groups and political representatives, and the hospital complaints procedure allows for this. It has been suggested that up to half of complaints about hospitals from both sexes concern the experiences of someone other than the complainant, usually a relative (Lloyd-Bostock & Mulcahy 1994). We argue in this chapter that it would be more appropriate to refer to complainant-centred systems.

The importance of non-patient complainant evaluations should not be underestimated. Friends or relatives may have a unique perspective on the service delivery process. They alone may know the true extent to which a patient's condition has deteriorated; that a nurse has been rude; that inadequate notice has been given of a patient's arrival home; that the seats in the waiting room are uncomfortable; or that the car park is always full. Not only this, they often have experience of the dissatisfaction which prompts the complaint. Research has demonstrated that complainants whose complaints concerned the experiences of another may not merely be acting as a conduit for the expression of another's grievance. Rather, they may be expressing their own dissatisfaction with the way their relative or friend had been treated (Lloyd-Bostock & Mulcahy 1994).

Complaints may be one way to facilitate patient-centred health care. They are one way for patients and others to give feedback which may be used to improve patient care. They are also a means to satisfy the patient populations' right to redress when something goes wrong. But a complainant-centred approach is not always the same as a patient-centred approach for three main reasons. First, individual complainants' needs are not unidimensional and may conflict with the collective interests of patients. Complainants are also part of a larger client group of patients or potential patients – consumers of health services. To this end, they have an interest not just in particular episodes of care but in the provision and quality of care more generally. As such, complainants may be viewed as proxies of a larger population of service users. Their needs may conflict with those of service users as a whole, with the result that a complaints system may be patient-centred without being complainant-centred, or complainant-centred without being patient-centred. Satisfying a complainant's demand to be put in a single sex ward, to have additional tests undertaken, or to be put higher up a waiting list may, for example, make overall provision of care less efficient, effective or equitable. Complainants are also part of a wider population of citizens and taxpayers who have an interest in general standards of fairness in the handling of complaints, as well as cost effective provision of health care.

Second, complainants may be atypical of patients in general. Meeting the interests of complainants may act against the interests of the patient population. A study conducted for the Department of Health by Mulcahy and Tritter found that formal complaints are representative of only certain types of dissatisfaction. Allegations about 'hotel' services were much more likely to emerge in formal complaints procedures than in their study of dissatisfied service users, whereas those allegations relating to management, policy and political issues tended to be underrepresented (Mulcahy & Tritter 1994).

Third, complaints procedures can clearly have a number of goals, not all of which appear to be centred on complainant needs. They can be used, amongst other things, for the early identification and management of potential medical negligence claims with a view to protecting the assets of the hospital; as managerial tools in the assessment of quality; as an opportunity to improve the image of the hospital; or as a dispute resolution tool. Not all of these goals are compatible. A system which aims to limit the financial liability of a hospital by early suppression of dissatisfaction may not, for example, serve to improve the image of the hospital or encourage full resolution of emerging disputes. Each hospital complaints procedure may have its own set of different priorities.

Whilst any one system may be criticized for not placing the complainants' interests first, the system cannot be properly evaluated until the extent to which it satisfies other, competing interests has also been fully understood. In addition, a number of different actors concerned about complainant needs, have different perspectives on how a complainant-centred approach could be adopted. This raises the issue of what goal we should be looking to, and whose standards should be used, when assessing whether the system is patient-centred.

The NHS hospital complaints system

The hospital complaints procedure appears to have two principal aims. First, it seeks to provide responses to, and redress of, citizen grievances. Second, it seeks to encourage the managerial monitoring of adverse incidents, and revision of practice or policy in response to them. The current system is governed by the Hospital Complaints Act 1985 and guidance issued under it. Under the Act health authorities are obliged to establish a formal complaints procedure. The most recent detailed guidelines are contained in a 1988 Circular, HC(88)37. According to these, each NHS unit must appoint a designated officer to investigate and respond to any complaint classified as formal. The Patient's Charter (DoH 1992) requires that all responses to formal complaints come from a senior manager.

If complainants are dissatisfied with the way the designated officer has responded to their complaint they can do one of two things, depending on what their dissatisfaction relates to. If the complaint concerns clinical aspects of care they can refer the matter to the regional director of public health, who is expected to arrange a meeting between the complainant and the staff involved. If the complaint remains unresolved the regional director can consider sending the matter to an independent professional review in which two consultants determine whether clinical judgment has been appropriately exercised. Alternatively, where complainants are still dissatisfied with the hospital's response, or with the way the health authority has handled the investigation, they can refer the matter to the Health Service Commissioner who has the power, where he sees fit, to initiate a full inquiry into the manner in which the complaint has been handled.

Reform of these procedures is imminent. In 1994 the government set up a committee under the chairmanship of Sir Alan Wilson to review current procedures. The committee recommended that the hospital complaints system be merged with that which operates for GPs and that appeals about complaints be heard by an independent committee with lay representatives (Department of Health 1994).

State mandated systems for redress of citizen grievances

Redress of citizen grievance has long been seen as a function of the state and it is to be expected that the state has an interest in the protection of the disputants' right to be heard. The interests of disputants can be protected by the state through legislation and policy which set standards to be applied in the resolution of disputes. The state's interest in the resolution of disputes can be understood in two contrasting ways. Traditionally it has been described in terms of citizen empowerment and civil liberties. As long ago as the Magna Carta the state guaranteed citizens the right to redress of their grievances. This approach assumes that the state gives prominence to the interests of its citizens and places value on the fair resolution of individuals' grievances. A more cynical view is that the state's interest is best understood in terms of the control that the central organs of the state exercise over its members by suppressing conflict that threatens the status quo and keeping people relatively passive by allowing some, albeit reduced, participation (Abel 1982).

One way to judge whether the complaints system is complainant-centred is to look to the standards imposed on dispute resolution mechanisms by the state. The extent to which there exists a comprehensive set of compatible criteria governing the handling of disputes by organs of the state has been questioned (Mulcahy & Tritter 1995). It is clear that there is actually very little design to our civil justice system and that its expansion and development has tended to be piecemeal and ad hoc rather than systematic (Harlow & Rawlings 1985). In the words of Lewis and Birkinshaw (1993):

> 'Justice is a hooray word. Everyone is in favour of it; governments take for granted that it is endemic in our system. When egregious instances of injustice occur, then they assume that these are instances of falling from a state of grace. Yet in a peculiarly British way, we are

not taken to sitting down and looking systematically at the whole of our political system.'

A major problem in specifying whether or not the hospital complaints system is a fair system is knowing the standards according to which it should be judged. Common sense suggests that it is in the public interest for any system of redress to be bound by the same core of public, coherent and mutually compatible principles. Despite this, reference in debate about civil justice is commonly made to a number of different established standards according to which systems for redress ought to operate; the doctrine of natural justice and procedural fairness are examples of these. More recently, the Citizen Charter Unit Complaints Task Force (1993) has specified 51 questions which organizations should use to evaluate their complaints systems. These relate key charter principles more directly to the handling of complaints across the public sector. They suggest that complaints systems should be simple and easy to use, speedy, allow for full and fair investigations, confidential and able to provide an effective response and appropriate redress.

It is difficult to assess the extent to which clear patterns emerge from any of these sets of criteria. To a large extent, analysis is hampered by such expansive concepts as 'fairness'. Moreover, the needs of the complainant may not coincide with general principles of dispute resolution. Whilst attention might be paid to disputant satisfaction, standards relating to the public resolution of disputes are not patient-centred in the sense that the interests of the complainant are put above those of other parties. The resolution of disputes in the NHS can, for instance, involve a choice between the competing arguments of actors involved in the dispute such as patient, doctor, manager. Indeed, adjudicatory models require this. In such cases, the complainant's interests may be just one of those to be taken into account. Not only does this mean that the resolution may not be complainant-centred, but that a certain amount of complainant dissatisfaction with process and outcome may be inevitable.

The organizational perspective

Whilst it could be argued that the state has an interest in overseeing the provision of redress systems and designing systems which are accessible, it is those working in the hospital sector who have the day to day task of enforcing standards, assessing needs and responding to criticisms and complaints. Managers are key actors in the provision of health care, and are increasingly being seen as agents of the patient population as a whole. As the person responsible for responding to complaints and facilitating improvements in service as a result of complaints, the manager occupies a pivotal role in the assessment of complainant and patient needs. As well as having a responsibility towards complainants, managers have a responsibility towards the local population, patients, doctors and other staff. In addition they will be concerned about the public image of the hospital and protection of its assets. The responsibilities are such that they may clash. A duty of candour to complainants may conflict with attention to procedural fairness for all the parties to the dispute.

Complaints and quality assurance

One area where there is minimal conflict is in the field of quality assurance. Not only does it place emphasis on the use of complaints as tools in the provision of better quality care, it reflects a sensitivity towards the altruistic motivations of many complainants. Alongside other indicators, such as patient satisfaction surveys, complaints can provide valuable warnings of a breakdown in service provision.

If complaints are to be of use in improving quality for all users it has been argued that they must be encouraged, and the implications of criticisms pursued and acted upon. Mulcahy and Lloyd-Bostock (1992), in their study of hospital complaints, found that complaints appeared to have an impact on future performance of the hospital in only 59 (14.7%) cases in their sample. In 24 (40.7%) of those cases this involved a review of procedures and policies and in 20 (33.9%) it involved an implementation of changes to procedures or policies. They discovered that in most cases 'investigations' of complaints consisted of copying the complainant's letter to staff under cover of a short note. These replies were then amalgamated into a latter of response.

The findings of this research suggest that managers tended to adopt a passive role, merely 'processing' complaints. Managers never requested additional information about allegations from complainants and rarely asked specific or further questions of members of staff who provided written responses to the complaint. The finding suggests that rather than valuing the information provided, managers place greater priority on processing complaints as quickly as possible. They are often more realistically cast in the role of clinicians' agent. This suggests that they may not be in a position to protect either the individual complainant or the collective needs of service users where those needs are in conflict with those of the person being complained about.

The role of hospital staff

Despite hospital staff being part of the provider organizations being complained about, their needs and approach may well be in conflict with those of both management and complainants. Staff may have an intimate relationship with patients and their relatives based on trust and a sense of vocation. Their emotional investment in the care process may be great. But staff can be seen as both agents of patients in assessing health care and even in encouraging complaints as well as the subjects of criticism when complaints are made. Their role may shift from carer and facilitator to antagonist. The approach of staff may differ according to how they view the complaints procedure. They may, for instance, see it as a system for resolution of a dispute in which both parties are heard and a decision made about the relative merits of their cases, or as a means of protecting their reputation. Alternatively, the management of grievances may be seen as an extension of the treatment role in which the carer has responsibility to ensure that the complainant ceases to feel concerned. The extent to which the complainant is seen as an adversary or in partnership with the carer will have a dramatic impact on the handling of the complaint and on the satisfaction with process and outcome.

The complainant perspective

Finally we come to consider the perspective of the most important person in judging whether or not a system is complainant-centred: the complainant. The interests of individual complainants cannot be assumed to be synonymous with either the state exercising its dispute resolution role, or the manager acting as the agent of the organization, the staff within the organization or the patient population as a whole. In this section we ask: Is the current system user friendly? What do complainants want? And are they satisfied?

User friendly complaints systems

A well structured procedure is of little use if service users do not know of its existence. Unfortunately, understanding the relationships between the various systems for redress in the NHS is notoriously difficult. Alongside the hospital complaints procedure already described, we find a separate legislative scheme for complaints relating to GPs, dentists, opticians and pharmacists; ambulance services; community care; and child protection. The current system does little to encourage complaints. Among other things guidelines require that information about how to complain is not to be displayed in hospital wards lest it encourage patients to make 'unfounded' or 'frivolous' complaints. Provision of a state sanctioned system does not guarantee compliance with mandated goals.

The Association of Community Health Councils has claimed that, in its members' experience, few health authorities are fully meeting their obligations under current guidelines to publicize their complaints procedures (ACHEW 1990). Instead of producing special leaflets encouraging feedback, many are said to rely on sections inserted into pre-existing patient information booklets. This not only makes the information less accessible, but it also means that those using out-patients, accident and emergency, and long-term residential care tend not to receive it. Lack of accessibility is further demonstrated by research. Prescott Clarke *et al.* (1988) found in a survey of patients in four health districts that only 5% of those questioned knew how to make a formal complaint. Interview data from another study showed that although complainants were aware of the existence of a hospital complaints machinery in 30% of cases, they had been aware of it prior to complaining in only 6% of cases (Lloyd-Bostock & Mulcahy 1994).

Accessible systems for appeal

Standards of accessibility require not only that complaints are easy to make but that they are easy to pursue if initial handling of the complaint leaves the complainant dissatisfied. It is clear from the description of the complaints system above that the type of appeal available is highly dependent on the type of allegation made, and that the classification of complaints as 'clinical' or 'nonclinical' is critical in determining the extent to which the medical profession controls this review. Neither avenue of 'appeal' from the initial response of the hospital manager can be described as easily accessible by service users. Although any complaints referred to the Health Service Commissioner will be considered by his office, few are in fact taken up for review since emphasis is placed on the thorough reconsideration of a few instances of complaint handling by hospitals. As far as clinical complaints are concerned, the procedure does allow for an independent professional review of the clinical aspects of the case by two independent consultants, but referral to a review is at the discretion of the regional director of public health and not available as of right. It seems unlikely that future reform of the system will allow appeals as of right.

In their study of 399 hospital complaints, Lloyd-Bostock and Mulcahy (1994) found that despite significant levels of dissatisfaction regarding the handling of their complaint, few complainants pursued their grievance beyond the first response from the hospital. Sixty-nine (16%) wrote a second letter to the hospital, and 18 wrote further letters, but the complaints were not taken beyond district level. In their sample there was no evidence that any of the cases studied were taken further through the formal complaints procedure to an independent professional review or the Health Service Commissioner. The possibility of referral to the Health Service Commissioner was raised in one case by the community health council but there was no evidence that it was pursued.

Understanding what complainants want

Complaints about hospital services are increasingly being seen as a way of facilitating client participation in the provision of care. One way to assess how best to respond to complaints is to be clear what it is that the complainant wants. This is not always an easy task. Some complaints have an obvious purpose. If someone complains that they have not been given treatment, it is probably safe to assume that they are complaining in order to get the situation remedied. However, many hospital complaints are not instrumental in this sense, and the goal or goals are not necessarily obvious in written accounts of dissatisfaction. In their analysis of 342 letters of complaint, Lloyd-Bostock and Mulcahy found that in 165 letters (48.2%) there was either no statement at all or only a 'vague' statement of what the complainant wanted.

Other statements of the response or action requested were grouped into three main categories. First, specific requests that something should be done to put matters right for this complainant, for instance that someone should be disciplined or an apology made (15.5% of letters). Second, that steps should be taken to put matters right to others in the future (19.9%). Third, requests relating to the provision of information about what has gone wrong (20.8%). The data suggests that the majority of complaints do not pose a great threat to the organisation or staff. Only seven (2%) of complainants in the sample wanted a member of staff punished and only nine (2.6%) wanted compensation, and the majority of these requests related to small amounts such as reimbursement of parking fines. In view of these findings, health care providers could usefully take steps to clarify what the complainant wants where this is not apparent. One way to achieve this might be to routinely consider whether a meeting with the complainant would facilitate an appropriate response to their grievance.

Complainant satisfaction

Another way to explore whether a system is complainant-centred is to measure complainant satisfaction with it and, in particular, whether a complainant wants what has been achieved. Regardless of what they wanted, Lloyd-Bostock and Mulcahy found significant levels of dissatisfaction with the way in which complaints were handled by hospitals. When asked to rate their satisfaction overall with the handling of their complaint on a ten-point scale, the average overall satisfaction rating was 4.8, with 58% giving a rating of 5 or less – i.e. more dissatisfied than satisfied. (Participants had been told that a score of 5 or less indicated that they were more dissatisfied than satisfied, and 6 or over that they were more satisfied than dissatisfied.)

It is often suggested that most complainants would be satisfied with an apology and Lloyd-Bostock and Mulcahy's analysis paid particular attention to this. Sixty-three per cent of letters of response contained some form of expression of regret (excluding condolences on a bereavement). But the mere use of words or phrases such as 'I am sorry' or 'I apologize' was not considered a full apology. Many of the apologies offered to complainants might on analysis be called incomplete or 'pseudoapologies' (Lloyd-Bostock 1993). They contained the word 'apology' 'apologies' 'sorry' or 'regret' but did not acknowledge that anything complaint-worthy had happened, or indicate a willingness to improve matters. What at first glance may seem to be an apology may not relate to the substance of the complaint at all, but rather be an expression of regret about something else; for example, 'I was sorry to learn of your husband's continued ill-health'; 'I was sorry to get your letter'; 'I am sorry that you felt you had to complain'.

Interviews with complainants confirmed that hospitals' replies frequently appeared defensive, and that the elements of a full apology related strongly to their satisfaction with the response. Thirty-six per cent rated the hospital as 'not at all' accepting responsibility for the event complained of; 57% rated the hospital as 'very much' or 'rather' trying to defend itself. Forty-one per cent said that they had been given an 'unsatisfactory explanation'.

During their analysis it became clear that it is important to complainants that their complaint be acknowledged and taken seriously, and that the hospital accept responsibility. It is particularly interesting to note the strong positive correlation between satisfaction and the complainant's belief that the hospital intended to 'improve things for the future'. This finding suggests that when complainants state that they are complaining in order to prevent others suffering in future, they genuinely wish for this and are not merely justifying their complaint with reference to altruistic goals. The finding also supports the proposition underlying the analysis of apologies offered by the authors, that if an apology is to fulfil its mitigating social function, it is important that the hospital give substance to its explanations and statements of remorse by conceding that matters are (or were) unsatisfactory and indicating its intention to take remedial action.

Conclusions

In this chapter we have attempted to highlight the conflicts which exist within the hospital complaints procedure. We have demonstrated the many ways in which responsibility for the provision of a complainant-centred system is shared between the state, hospital managers and staff. In addition we have argued that the needs of complainants are often in conflict with others whose views ought to be considered. In the provision of patient-centred health care it is particularly important to be aware of the extent to which the interests of collective patient population conflict with those of individual complainants.

At the very least, complaints provide a detection system to help improve patient care. If information about defects in the system is to be maximized, patients and relatives need to be encouraged to use the system. Better publicity is needed so that service users are aware of the complaints system. Second, the procedure should seriously address, in the case of every complaint, the issue of what can be learnt or how patient care can be improved. Adopting this stance should help to counteract the types of defensive response we have highlighted. But the system should not just be designed with organisational improvement in mind. It should also provide adequate ways of redressing individual grievances. In order to be complainant-centred the procedure should:

- clarify what the complainant wants;
- offer a remedy which is appropriate for that complainant.

With the recent publication of the Wilson Committee review of NHS complaints procedures (DoH 1994), the issue of how complainant-centred NHS complaints systems are, has become a particular interest of policy makers. As the perspectives of complainants, state, manager, clinicians and other staff are each presented, a key issue to be resolved will be whether a reformed procedure will adopt a model where the priority is to establish the accuracy of the complainant's claims, or whether the handling of complaints is to be seen as part of a service provision which aims to satisfy its users. Whilst the former would recognize the competing needs of both the complainant and the subject of the complaint, the latter would prioritize those needs in favour of the complainant.

Whether or not the issue is recognized or addressed, what becomes apparent from a review of the present system is that there is a need to improve accessibility, the quality of responses and the use made of some complaints as indicators of bad quality. In the words of the Wilson Committee (DoH 1994):

> 'People generally have considerable trust in the services the NHS provides. They expect – and usually receive – care of the highest quality, and they offer gratitude and praise freely as a result. When they believe there is something wrong, it is by no means easy for them to raise their concerns. They are not in a powerful position and may feel vulnerable. The response they get when they make a complaint is a fundamental test of the NHS as a public service.'

The patient-centred model has much to offer as complaints systems in the NHS are reviewed and refocused. But whilst the goal of patient-centred care is the subject of consensus, the goal of complainant-centred systems is still the subject of debate.

Reading guide

Much of what has been written on complaints in the NHS is descriptive and policy oriented. A good general review of criticisms of the current procedures is contained in *Being Heard* (DoH 1994). This also suggests a number of options for change. The major empirical studies of the system have been reported by Allsop (1994) in *Two sides to every story: complainant's and doctor's perspectives in disputes about medical care in a general practice setting*, by Donaldson and Cavanagh (1992) in *Clinical complaints and their handling: a time for a change*, by Lloyd-Bostock and Mulcahy (1994) in *The social psychology of making and responding to hospital complaints: an account model of complaint processes*, and by Mulcahy and Lloyd-Bostock (1994) in *Managers as third party dispute handlers in complaints about hospitals*. In addition, an attempt has been made to look at complaints in the context of patient dissatisfaction, by Mulcahy and Tritter (1994) in *Hidden depths*, of quality assurance by Mulcahy and Lloyd-Bostock (1992) in *Complaining – what's the use?*, and finally in the context of risk management by Allsop and Mulcahy (in press) in *Dealing with clinical complaints*.

References

Abel, R. (1982) The contradictions of informal justice. In: *The Politics of Informal Justice.* Academic Press, New York.

ACHEW (1990) *National Health Service Complaints Procedures.* Association of Community Health Councils for England and Wales, London.

Allsop, J. (1994) Two sides to every story: complainant's and doctor's perspectives in disputes about medical care in a general practice setting. *Law and Policy,* **16**(2), 149–84.

Allsop, J. & Mulcahy, L. (in press) Dealing with clinical complaints. In: *Clinical Risks* (ed. C. Vincent). BMJ Publications, London.

Citizens' Charter Unit Complaints Task Force (1993) *Effective Complaints Systems: Principles and Checklist.* HMSO, London.

Complaints Task Force (1993) *Effective Complaint Handling: Principles and Check List,* Citizen's Charter Unit. HMSO, London.

DoH (1992). *The Patient's Charter.* HMSO, London.

DoH (1994) *Being Heard – The Report of the Review Committee on NHS Complaints Procedures.* HMSO, London.

Donaldson, L. & Cavanagh, J. (1992) Clinical complaints and their handling: a time for a change. *Quality in Health Care,* March.

Harlow, C. & Rawlings, R. (1985) *Law and Adminstration.* Weidenfield & Nicholson, London.

Lewis, N. & Birkinshaw, P. (1993) *When Citizens Complain.* Open University Press, Buckingham.

Lloyd-Bostock, S. (1993) Attributions of cause and responsibility as social phenomena. In: *Attribution Theory and Research: Conceptual Developmental and Social Dimensions* (eds J.M.F. Jaspars, F.D. Fincham & M. Hewstone). Academic Press, New York.

Lloyd-Bostock, S. & Mulcahy, L. (1994) The social psychology of making and responding to hospital complaints: an account model of complaint processes. *Law and Policy,* **16**(2), 123–47.

Mulcahy, L. & Lloyd-Bostock, S. (1992) Complaining – what's the use? In: *Quality and Regulation in Healthcare* (eds R. Dingwall & P. Fenn). Routledge, London.

Mulcahy, L. & Lloyd-Bostock (1994) Managers as third party dispute handlers in complaints about hospitals. *Law and Policy,* **16**(2), 185–208.

Mulcahy, L. & Tritter, J. (1994) Hidden Depths. *Health Services Journal,* July, pp. 24–6.

Mulcahy, L. & Tritter, J. (1995) Rhetoric or redress? The place of the Citizen's Charter in the civil justice system. In: *Citizen Empowerment in the New Public Sector* (ed. C. Willett). Elgar Press, London.

Prescott-Clarke, P. Brooks, T. & Machray, C. (1988) *Focus on Health Care – A Survey of the Public in Four Districts.*Royal Institute of Public Administration and Social Community Planning Research, London.

Commentary on Chapter 14

Maeve Ennis

The issues raised in the excellent chapter by Mulcahy and Lloyd-Bostock highlight the conflict inherent in the current complaints procedure, where the interests of the individual complainant may not be the interests of the patient population as a whole or the interests of those providing health care, be they managers, doctors or other health care workers. The chapter also demonstrates the often adversarial nature of the complaints procedure and the frequently defensive response of the providers.

I wish to respond from the perspective of my own work in underlying causes of medical accidents (Vincent *et al.* 1993) and work which has looked at cases where the complaints procedure has failed or been by-passed and litigation has ensued (Ennis & Vincent 1990; Ennis *et al.* 1991; Vincent *et al.* 1994).

The very term patient-centred health care would suggest a system of health care provision that is run for the benefit of patients, both individually and collectively. Inherent in such a system would be the notion that where patients or those acting for them have a grievance, these grievances would be dealt with speedily and fairly and that the information gained from this process would be used to ensure that whenever possible such things would never happen again. Sadly, as Mulcahy and Lloyd-Bostock have shown, this is seldom the case. Where complaints could be used to improve standards of care they found managers 'tended to adopt a passive role' and that they are often cast in the role of 'clinicians' agent', failing to inform patients on how to express grievances or complain, and when complaints are made responding in a defensive and adversarial manner. This is despite the fact that few complainants want either a member of staff punished or compensation, the majority just wishing that such things would not happen again in the future.

These findings are somewhat mirrored in work which has looked at cases that have come to litigation (Ennis & Vincent 1990; Vincent *et al.* 1994). Claims for compensation and complaints are not the same. Very few complaints proceeded to claims and many of those who seek redress through litigation by-pass the complaints procedure altogether. Why patients go to court in the first instance is not entirely clear, but it may be an expression of the depth of their anger, or even an ignorance of the complaints procedure. It may be that the majority of claims, unlike complaints, concern adverse clinical incidents in which a patient has been injured or died because of their treatment, and patients or their agents feel that the seriousness of the matter needs a wider hearing than that offered by the complaints procedures.

However, many of the points expressed by complainants – such as lack of provision of an apology and statement of accountability when things go wrong, a wish that it should not happen to others in the future, and the provision of information about what happened – are also expressed by those taking legal action. Obviously in some cases of litigation a need for compensation may be the main reason for bringing the claim; for example, if someone is injured, particularly a child, the financial burden of care over a long period of time can be great. But even in these cases the motivation for bringing a claim may not be exclusively financial but may in fact be determined by the way the incident was handled by staff concerned in the first place.

In our study of obstetric accidents (Ennis & Vincent 1990) we found that while many claimants had a need for financial compensation, one of the overriding reasons for suing a health authority or doctor was the need to find out how they or their baby was injured or died, and in the case of injury, what the long term effects were likely to be. Many reported that it was only through bringing a law suit that they had access to vital information. This was of course prior to the Access to Health Records Act (HMSO 1990), but even with this access to their medical records many did not find the explanation they needed as records were sometimes missing and often incomplete – in one case the actual birth was not recorded – and when the case came to court, sometimes years later, hospital staff memory of the incident was often vague. In some of these cases a possible explanation of what happened came, not from the hospital or staff concerned, but from an independent expert. Whether or not all these patients would have sued had they had this explanation in the first place is not known.

A study by Vincent *et al.* found that even when an explanation was given, many claimants were still dissatisfied. Less than 40% felt that the explanations were given in a sympathetic manner and the majority were felt to be 'unclear, inaccurate and lacking information'; responsibility for what happened was accepted in only 13% of cases and a full or partial apology offered in only 15% of cases. Of the 227 cases taking legal action, looked at in this study, a formal enquiry was instituted on only 19 (8%) of occasions (Vincent *et al.* 1994).

This study suggests that, at least in these cases, the major reasons for litigation were standards of care, explanation, accountability and compensation. It is interesting to note that 41% of these claimants stated that had something been offered at an earlier stage (explanation, compensation, investigation, correction of mistake) they would not have proceeded to litigation (Vincent *et al.* 1994); so it would appear that at least some patients are using litigation as an extension of the complaints procedure.

Mulcahy and Lloyd-Bostock suggest that complainants should be viewed as proxies of a larger population of service users who have an interest in the provision and quality of care, and this must also be true of those who bring claims. However, in the case of claimants it would appear that in a service with limited financial resources, a claim for financial compensation from an individual must be in conflict with the needs of service users as a whole. The cost of settling claims in the mid 1980s is £125m a year, 2.6% of the NHS budget (Hickey, pers. comm.). Money to pay claims is money diverted from other areas of the service. From this it could be argued that the claims procedure is patient-centred. However, this is not to argue that it is necessarily in anyone's best interest for patients to go to litigation. A patient who has suffered injury as a consequence of medical treatment may be severely trau-matized by the incident. Many suffer severe psychological distress for many years afterwards, a distress that is exacerbated by the litigation process. Doctors may also suffer psychological distress and in some cases it can lead to maladaptive behaviour towards patients (Ennis & Vincent 1994); as has been shown earlier the financial cost to the service as a whole is considerable.

It would seem that complaints and litigation could be instruments in improving the quality of care. Mulcahy and Lloyd-Bostock found this not to be the case and other findings were that litigation and fear of litigation led to defensive medicine (Ennis *et al.* 1991; Harvard Medical Practice Study 1990).

This leads to the final area I wish to discuss: the adversarial nature of both the claims procedure and litigation. The terms 'blame' and 'responsibility' appear to be muddled in the eyes of hospital managers and doctors. When something goes wrong, very often no one person is at fault and in the case of medical accidents it is often a series of minor incidents that lead to a negative outcome for the patient. But too often the organizational response to claims and litigation is that someone must be to blame and therefore their responsibility is to defend this individual rather than look at the complaint/claim in a more global manner. It is, for example, useless to blame junior doctors for acting beyond their competence when, because of staff shortages, no senior was available or their training was inadequate. In a very limited sense the junior is to 'blame' for carrying out the procedure, but overall responsibility does not lie with him/her but at a higher level and this must be recognized and responded to in a responsible manner which satisfies all parties.

I hope that in this response to Mulcahy and Lloyd-Bostock I have demonstrated that the need of litigants and complainants are little different and that both groups would benefit from a patient-centred complaints procedure. Perhaps if we had a better patient-centred model for complaints we would not need litigation.

References

Access to Health Records Act (1990). HMSO, London.

Ennis, M. & Vincent, C. (1990) Obstetric accidents: a review of 64 cases. *British Medical Journal*, **300**, 26 May, 1365–7.

Ennis, M., Clark, A. & Grudzinskas, J. (1991) Change in obstetric practice in response to fear of litigation in the British Isles. *The Lancet*, **338**, 616–18.

Harvard Medical Practice Study (1990) *Patients, doctors and lawyers: medical injury, malpractice litigation, and patient compensation in New York.* Report of the Harvard Medical Practice Study. Harvard University Press, Cambridge.

Vincent, C., Ennis, M. & Audley, R. (eds) (1993) *Medical Accidents.* Oxford University Press, Oxford.

Vincent, C., Young, M. & Phillips, A. (1994) Why do people sue doctors? A study of patients and relatives taking legal action. *The Lancet*, **343**, 25 June.

15 ◆ Patient-Centred Approaches to the Evaluation of Health Care

Ray Fitzpatrick

Two parallel and possibly mutually supportive rhetorics have emerged in health care policy in recent years. One emphasizes the role and value of patient-centred approaches to the provision of care. The second emphasizes the role and value of the patient in the evaluation of care. Both rhetorics have a great deal of persuasiveness in them and have prompted considerable activities to change health care services in directions that are more patient-centred in their delivery and, as a consequence, more favourably received by patients as reflected in their views on outcomes.

The objective of this chapter is to raise some questions about patient-centred outcome measures and then ask the question whether current measures are appropriate to patient-centred care. The first part of the chapter reviews a range of constructs and measures that have been developed to put patients' experiences to the fore. They are referred to here, as in most discussions, as quality of life measures, although they are much more limited in range than this term implies. Their significance for discussions of patient-centred care is that they represent the results of considerable efforts by many researchers to focus on the patients' experiences of their health problems. These measures are viewed as sufficiently important to constitute a potential revolution in health care as they require that patients' values become central in the evaluation and, hence, future development of health services (Ellwood 1988; Fitzpatrick & Albrecht 1994).

Conceptual uncertainties

The family of measures that attempt to capture patients' experiences in terms of so-called quality of life is not based on elaborate conceptual or theoretical analysis. Overviews of the field repeatedly emphasize how ill-defined, limited in scope and poorly measured are the instruments used in the vast majority of medical studies purporting to include quality of life (Aaronson 1989; Fallowfield 1989; Guyatt *et al.* 1989; Najman & Levine 1981; Schumacher *et al.* 1991). There have nevertheless been some attempts to produce a coherent and comprehensive definition of quality of life that would be relevant to health care. However, they are notable mainly for their heterogeneity. Definitions variously emphasize the capacity of individuals to realize their life plans; the ability of patients to manage their lives as they evaluate them; the difference between reality and expectations; the sum of the individual's health, subjective wellbeing and welfare; a composite of the ability to perform everyday activities, satisfaction with functioning, and satisfaction with the control of disease (Dimenas *et al.* 1990; Fowlie & Berkeley 1987; Gotay & Moore 1992).

One review of questionnaire-based quality of life measures in health care argues that most instruments contain items that can be placed under one or more of the following dimensions: emotional well-being, spirituality, sexuality, social functioning, family life, occupational functioning, communication, eating, functional ability, physical status, treatment satisfaction, future orientation and global ratings of health or life satisfaction (Cella & Tulsky 1990). The majority of instruments can be described by an even smaller list of dimensions: emotional status, physical function, social functioning and symptoms (Fitzpatrick *et al.* 1992). It is frequently observed that measures tend to focus exclusively on the patient and do not take account of the quality of life of family, carers or the community of the patient (Anderson & Bury 1988; Jenkins 1992). It is common to focus on health-related quality of life since broader aspects of the construct are not relevant to health care. However it is not clear how to identify precisely this subset of the broader range of personal experience.

How patients define quality of life

A small number of studies have asked patients to say directly what they regard as the most important dimensions of quality of life. Study designs vary sufficiently to make it hard to generalize from results. However, it is clear that patients' wellbeing incorporates a wider range of factors than symptoms. In studies of patients with a variety of major health problems, family relationships in particular are cited as either most important or amongst the most important components of quality of life (Kreitler *et al.* 1993; McGee *et al.* 1991; O'Boyle *et al.* 1992; Sutherland *et al.* 1990). Patients may also report that their social life, leisure activities or ability to maintain independence are just as important influences upon quality of life as symptoms or health problems (Kreitler *et al.* 1993; O'Boyle *et al.* 1992; Sutherland *et al.* 1990).

Does illness influence quality of life?

In view of the evidence that patients report a wide range of factors as relevant to their quality of life, it is worth considering how close the relationship is between, on the one hand, disease and illness and, on the other hand, quality of life and wellbeing. One of the largest studies to date has been the Medical Outcomes Study in which a large number of patients with a number of different chronic health problems completed a quality of life (QOL) instrument in relation to a visit to their doctor (Stewart *et al.* 1989). Patients with a prior heart attack, or with congestive cardiac failure, diabetes, arthritis, gastrointestinal or chronic lung problems, had poorer scores than a healthy comparison group recruited from the general population, especially for performance of physical activities, work and housework.

It is striking that patients with chronic health problems also experienced significantly poorer scores for emotional wellbeing compared with the healthy controls, but the differences were not nearly so great as for more physical dimensions. Other studies using different instruments also indicate greater differences in QOL between chronically ill and well individuals for more physical aspects of wellbeing, and only small differences for psychological wellbeing (Brazier *et al.* 1992; Stewart *et al.* 1989). In one widely cited study, patients with either arthritis, diabetes, cancer, renal disease or various dermatological disorders were compared to well individuals on standardized psychological wellbeing scales. No differences were found in comparisons with well individuals (Cassileth *et al.* 1984).

In such studies, effects of chronic illness on QOL are less apparent with regard to psychological wellbeing than for more physical aspects of QOL. In several studies patients with serious health problems have rated their quality of life as favourably as have healthy comparison groups (Kreitler *et al.* 1993; McGee *et al.* 1991; O'Boyle *et al.* 1992). Health problems may challenge individuals' general sense of wellbeing to a lesser extent than might be expected.

Disease severity and quality of life

In several comparative studies it has been noted that the majority of variance in QOL is unexplained by means of disease category (Stewart *et al.* 1989; Viney & Westbrook 1981). Differences in QOL between illnesses may be less marked because underlying disease processes vary in severity, both between individuals and over time. Studies of a wide range of health problems have shown that increased disease severity is associated with poorer QOL (Deyo *et al.* 1982; Guyatt *et al.* 1987; Kaplan *et al.* 1989; Regan *et al.* 1991; Rudick *et al.* 1992).

However, it is striking that the size of the correlation between disease severity and QOL variables tends to be quite modest, particularly with regard to components such as psychological wellbeing. In the majority of the studies cited above very little of the variance in QOL is explained by conventional measures of disease severity. Indeed in a few studies the correlations may actually be positive, with more severely ill patients expressing more favourable QOL (Brown *et al.* 1981; Evans 1991).

Mediating factors

Much of the literature on patients' experiences of health and illness is excessively static and fails to capture the coping strategies and processes of adjustment that undoubtedly diminish the impact of disease processes on patient wellbeing (Deyo *et al.* 1982; Newman *et al.* 1989). In some conditions, such as some cancers, there may be a U-shaped relationship, with wellbeing diminished on learning the diagnosis and during later stages of terminal care, but a positive process of adaptation between these points (Fallowfield & Clark 1991; Silberfarb *et al.* 1980). For many chronic illnesses there may be a more cyclical process of adaptation and diminished wellbeing following severe acute exacerbations of disease (Jenkins 1992). According to the striking evidence of Cassileth and colleagues (1984), however, the process of positive adaptation over time is linear, direct and consistent across a wide range of diseases. Processes invoked to explain such evidence include denial, goal-restructuring, minimization of disease consequences, and changing reference groups.

The obverse of such positive coping strategies are a range of cognitive and emotional responses to illness which emphasize helplessness and catastrophizing. Such responses are related to poorer self assessment of quality of life (Affleck *et al.* 1987; Fitzpatrick *et al.* 1989). At worst, patients with chronic illness who also experience depression view their quality of life, health status and wellbeing more negatively than would be predicted by disease state (Barsky *et al.* 1992; Sensky & Catalan 1992; Wells *et al.* 1989).

The judgements of observers

One important justification for the development of structured measures of patients' wellbeing is the evidence that health professionals are often not very good at judging the subjective experiences of their patients. In studies of a diverse range of patient groups, it has been shown that physicians' ratings of patients' quality of life and related constructs such as psychological wellbeing agree only moderately with those of the patients whom they assess (Pearlman & Uhlmann 1988; Schag *et al.* 1984; Slevin *et al.* 1988). Usually health professionals' judgements are more negative than those of their patients (Spitzer *et al.* 1981; Sprangers & Aaronson 1992). The differences are greater for more subjective aspects of quality of life compared with dimensions that may be more visible such as functional status (Sprangers & Aaronson 1992; Teske *et al.* 1983; Uhlmann & Pearlman 1991).

Quality of life as utilities

The subject of quality of life in health care is now dominated by a quite different tradition of research concerned with quality adjusted life years (QALYs). QALYs are a method of expressing benefits of health care in terms of survival adjusted for quality of life. Much of the original work in this field did not set out explicitly to assess quality of life per se, referring instead to valuations (Rosser & Kind 1976) or utilities (Sackett & Torrance 1978) of different health states. Such terms make it clear that the objective is primarily to obtain a set of values for all states of health including death. A number of methods have now been developed whereby panels of experimental respondents may be encouraged to provide their judgements of the severity or desirability of varying states of ill-health: standard gamble, time-trade-off, category scaling, magnitude estimation, equivalence and willingness to pay. Although varying in details, each of these methods relies on the judgements made by individuals asked to imagine various health states; whereas the work reviewed above focuses directly on the experiences of those with a health problem.

Although one may do an injustice to nuances of difference between studies of health utilities, there are clear tendencies identifiable in a number of studies obtained from samples from diverse western societies (Kaplan & Anderson 1988; Nord 1991; Williams & Kind 1992). Individuals imagine different health states to vary considerably in terms of quality of life. States of ill-health involving substantial disability are considered quite undesirable by experimental panels and therefore attract low quality of life scores. Moreover panels regard physical and psychological function to be equally important influences on utilities.

The contrast with studies of patients directly experiencing various health problems should be clear. Patients with direct experience of ill-health may suffer varying degrees of impairment and disability arising from their health problems, but commonly respond in positive terms regarding emotional wellbeing and quality of life. Experimental panels required instead to express preferences for different health states, emphasize the undesirability of health states involving poor physical function. Differences between the two approaches are not at all difficult to explain. There is now a reasonably substantial literature, particularly in psychology, to explain why individuals are not good judges of the actual rather than imagined desirability of different states, so that, in the current case, they make erroneous judgements of the quality of life of the ill (Kahneman & Varey 1991). Individuals appear to have very little insight into how to predict future preferences. They have little insight into the pervasive effects of habituation to the widest range of perceptual stimuli, not just health states. Moreover they are unaware of the contextual, comparative and relative nature of wellbeing.

It is clear from such evidence that there is a considerable amount of progress still needed before it can be said that patient-based measures of outcome in the QALYs and utilities field fully incorporate actual patients' experiences. The value to patients of health care may well systematically differ from the utilities derived from experimental panels. This is an important problem because evaluations of the benefits obtained from health care increasingly draw on QALY-type calculations to estimate benefits. Experimentally derived estimates of utilities tend to have a greater influence on such analyses that patients' own direct judgements.

There are a number of other objections to the use of QALYs to evaluate health care and they have been well rehearsed elsewhere (Smith 1987; Carr-Hill 1989). Methodological problems include whether QALYs adequately describe the range of health states; discrepancies between methods of eliciting values; possible framing effects upon values; and evidence of social variation in valuations. Practical problems include the lack of appropriate evidence regarding survival and quality of life for most interventions, and profound doubts about the public acceptability of QALY-based decisions. Ethical problems arise from the application of utilitarian as opposed to egalitarian or needs-based principles to resource allocation. However, the issue that is particularly pertinent to the context of patient-centred care concerns the appropriateness of QALY-type approaches to the evaluation of health care.

The functions of health care

QALYs are intended to assess the impact of health services upon survival and quality of life, two undoubtedly central objectives. However, health care fulfils a number of functions besides improving health status in terms of survival and quality of life; for example, reassurance, reduction of uncertainty, empathy and social support. Sometimes these functions will have impact upon health; for example, patients who feel that their doctor has made an effort to understand their problems may experience greater symptomatic improvement (Fitzpatrick *et al.* 1983; Headache Study Group of University of Western Ontario 1986), and doctors who increase the patient's sense of control over symptoms may have a favourable impact upon underlying health problems (Kaplan *et al.* 1989). Modest efforts to convey support towards patients may also have effects upon health status (Weinberger *et al.* 1986), and small amounts of additional information can reduce patients' discomfort and increase the speed of postsurgical recovery (Egbert *et al.* 1964). In addition, support, reassurance and enhancing control may improve adherence to advice (Kaplan *et al.* 1989).

Such direct therapeutic benefits of patient-centred approaches to health care, however, are unlikely to be consistently substantial and sufficient to register in QALY-type measures. More importantly, the intended purpose of functions such as empowering, confiding, reassuring, is not to influence health status but to meet a human need for a sense of control, empathy from others and reassurance. For various reasons advocates of the QALY-type approach would argue for the primacy of survival and quality of life outcomes to evaluate health care, with the result that other functions are not recognized. These various arguments are not well articulated and need to be drawn out for more explicit attention.

One line is that these other functions of health care are more vague and too difficult to measure (McGuire *et al.* 1988). It is therefore methodologically hard to incorporate them in cost–utility analyses. This is the weakest argument. Measures of constructs such as social support and sense of control are as psychometrically robust as those involved in QALYs and have as long a history of development (Lefcourt 1981; Orth-Gomer & Uden 1987). All such concepts, whether quality of life or social support, refer to subjective experiences that may be measured with more or less accuracy. The various personal skills involved in providing appropriate advice, empathy, support and reassurance are recognized by patients and reflected in measures of patient satisfaction (Fitzpatrick 1993).

A second objection to the expansion of dimensions of outcome beyond matters of survival and quality of life is that reassurance, support and other patient-centred actions are less to do with health (Mooney 1992). Outcomes should, according to this argument, be confined to those functions relevant to health care and health status. This argument is also weak. To regard functions such as reassurance and social support as less relevant to health is arbitrarily to redefine into limbo the activities of most of primary care and much of hospital care.

Another argument used is that reassurance and information giving, for example, are processes rather than outcomes of care (Williams & Kind 1992). This too suggests unhelpful semantic redefinition. These aspects are just as much outcomes as are reduced pain or depression.

The most powerful argument in defence of the supremacy of QALYs amongst outcomes is that any system that shifted its priorities to encompass a wider range of outcomes beyond QALYs thereby has serious consequences. As Williams and Kind (1992) graphically put it:

> 'If these alternative positions are indeed accepted by the general public as important additional objectives of the NHS, it should be recognized that their acceptance implies that the overall health of the population will be worse than it need have been. People on average will both die sooner and suffer more than they need have done.'

Williams and Kind put bluntly the trade-offs that may be required in terms of resource allocation when health care interventions which address the wider functions of health care receive resources at the expense of life saving services. There is an implied appeal to utilitarian principles in the stark statement of consequences. Society would be electing to make less than maximal use of its scarce resources by financing supportive care at the expense of life saving interventions.

Some would agree with this analysis but defend resource allocation to the wider functions of health care by appeal to other moral principles. Thus patients who receive palliative or supportive care, and do not derive benefits from QALYs as currently defined, ought to be cared for because of ethical principles which are as valid as utilitarianism. Thus patients deserve care on the basis of egalitarianism – every individual has some equal right to care (Potts 1992). Equally patients deserve care on the basis of either need, desert or compassion (Hope *et al.* 1993). According to such lines of argument it is conceded that many caring functions of health services cannot be defended on utilitarian grounds, and other equally valid moral criteria for resource allocation may need to be invoked. However it needs to be considered whether caring cannot also be defended in the utilitarian terms defined by QALYs.

The benefits of caring

Cost utility analyses are concerned particularly with assessing in comparative terms the benefits of different interventions. When results of such analyses are used in resource allocation decisions it is the relative value of different benefits in different treatments that is of concern. At present, benefits, and to a large extent relative values of benefits, are very indirectly assessed in QALY-type methods via judgements of panels imagining values of health states. Patients' perceptions of the benefits of services as direct recipients are filtered into measurement systems to the extent that benefits conform with externally defined criteria such as changes in distress and disability. Values of such benefits are further removed from those of patients by virtue of being determined by estimates of values directly derived from panels. Were perceived benefits of interventions to be more directly assessed by patients, a fuller range of factors would be included by patients; whether they were reassured or felt more in control of their symptoms as well as whether quality of life more narrowly defined was improved. To the extent that personal satisfactions of health care goals are the intended ingredients of utility analyses, it seems arbitrary in the extreme to include only a subset. Whether patients experience, for example, dignity, reassurance or sense of control may well, for some health care problems, figure quite highly in the set of personal goals and preferences, with survival and aspects of quality of life such as disability considered less important.

It may be objected that it would be a retrograde step if resource allocation for health care were to attempt to take account of subjective benefits such as dignity and reassurance in addition to the outcomes of survival and quality of life narrowly defined. Patients may experience such nonspecific benefits from many health care interventions which, from the balance of available evidence, we might consider ineffective and less deserving of resources. However, if two conditions are met, this objection is less cogent. First, both parties in any given health care intervention – patients and providers – must agree about whether provision of functions such as support or empathy is a major goal rather than a side-benefit of other more specific outcomes. Thus support and empathy should not be the most salient outcome measure if the goals of both parties are to replace a damaged hip, or reduce chest pain, but might be fundamental in the context of palliative care.

The second requirement is that it is demonstrated with evidence, rather than assumed, that support or other caring functions do have a significant impact on patients' perceptions of support. If these two conditions are met, it would seem that there are many forms of health care which do not significantly affect survival and health-related quality of life of the kind emphasized in QALYs, but which might nevertheless be expected to produce favourable impacts that are of importance in utilitarian terms.

This leads to the inevitable conclusion that patient-centred care, whether it is defended by appeal to utilitarianism or in terms of needs, will have to operationalize the relationships between components of the processes of care and the specific dimensions of outcome. The onus is upon us to identify the benefits that patients undoubtedly do experience from patient-centred care that are not detected by the currently used measures of outcome (Albrecht & Fitzpatrick 1994). By this means a health care system that is truly patient-centred will emerge.

Reading guide

Albrecht, G. & Fitzpatrick, R. (eds) (1994) *Quality of Life in Health Care.* JAI Press, Greenwich, Connecticut.

Anderson, R. & Bury, M. (1988) *Living with Chronic Illness.* Unwin Hyman, London.

Hopkins, A. (ed.) (1992) *Measures of the Quality of Life.* Royal College of Physicians, London.

Nordenfelt, E. (ed.) (1994) *Concepts and Measurement of Quality of Life in Health Care.* Kluwer Academic Press, Dordrecht.

References

Aaronson, N. (1989) Quality of life assessment in clinical trials: methodological issues. *Controlled Clinical Trials*, **10**, 195S–208S.

Affleck, G., Tennen, H., Pfeiffer, C. & Fifield, J. (1987) Appraisals of control and predictability in adapting to a chronic disease. *Journal of Personality and Social Psychology*, **53**, 273–9.

Albrecht, G. & Fitzpatrick, R. (eds) (1994) *Quality of Life in Health Care.* JAI Press, Greenwich, Connecticut.

Anderson, R. & Bury, M. (eds) (1988) *Living with Chronic Illness.* Unwin Hyman, London.

Barsky, A., Cleary, P. & Klerman, G. (1992) Determinants of perceived health status in medical outpatients. *Social Science and Medicine*, **34**, 1147–54.

Brazier, J., Harper, R., Jones, N. *et al.* (1992) Validating the SF-36 health survey questionnaire: new outcome measure for primary care. *British Medical Journal*, **305**, 160–4.

Brown, J., Rawlinson, M. & Hilles, N. (1981) Life satisfaction and chronic disease: exploration of a theoretical model. *Medical Care*, **19**, 1136–46.

Carr-Hill, R. (1989) Assumptions of the QALY procedure. *Social Science and Medicine*, **29**, 469–77.

Cassileth, B., Lusk, E., Strouse, T. *et al.* (1984) Psychosocial status in chronic illness: a comparative analysis of six diagnostic groups. *New England Journal of Medicine*, **311**, 506–11.

Cella, D. & Tulsky, D. (1990) Measuring quality of life today: methodological aspects. *Oncology*, **4**, 29–38.

Deyo, R, Inui, T., Leininger, J. & Overman, S. (1982) Physical and psychosocial function in rheumatoid arthritis. *Archives of Internal Medicine*, **142**, 879–82.

Dimenas, E., Dahlof, C., Jern, S. & Wiklund, I. (1990) Defining quality of life in medicine. *Scandinavian Journal of Health Care*, Suppl. 1, 7–10.

Egbert, L., Battit, G., Welsh, C. & Bartlett, M. (1964) Reduction of post-operative pain by encouragement and instructions of patients: a study of doctor–patient rapport. *New England Journal of Medicine*, **270**, 823–7.

Ellwood, P. (1988) Shattuck lecture – outcomes management. *New England Journal of Medicine*, **318**, 1549–56.

Evans, R. (1991) Quality of life. *The Lancet*, **338**, 636.

Fallowfield, L. (1989) *The Quality of Life*. Souvenir, London.

Fallowfield, L. & Clark, A. (1991) *Breast Cancer*. Routledge, London.

Fitzpatrick, R. (1993) Scope and measurement of patient satisfaction. In: Measurement of Patients' Satisfaction With Their Care. (eds R. Fitzpatrick & A. Hopkins), pp. 1–17. Royal College of Physicians, London.

Fitzpatrick, R. & Albrecht, G. (1994) The plausibility of quality of life measures in different domains of health care. In: *Concepts and Measurement of Quality of Life in Health Care* (ed. L. Nordenfelt), pp. 201–28. Kluwer Academic Publishers, Dordrecht.

Fitzpatrick, R., Hopkins, A. & Harvard-Watts, O. (1983) Social dimensions of healing: a longitudinal study of outcomes of medical management of headaches. *Social Science and Medicine*, **17**, 501–10.

Fitzpatrick, R., Newman, S., Lamb, R. & Shipley, M. (1989) Helplessness and control in rheumatoid arthritis. *International Journal of Health Sciences*, **1**, 17–23.

Fitzpatrick, R., Fletcher, A., Gore, S. *et al.* (1992) Quality of life measures in health care. I: Applications and issues in assessment. *British Medical Journal*, **305**, 1074–7.

Fowlie, M. & Berkeley, J. (1987) Quality of life: a review of the literature. *Family Practice*, **4**, 226–34.

Gotay, C. & Moore, T. (1992) Assessing quality of life in head and neck cancer. *Quality of Life Research*, **1**, 5–18.

Guyatt, G., Berman, L., Townsend, M. *et al.* (1987) A measure of quality of life for clinical trials in chronic lung disease. *Thorax*, **42**, 773–7.

Guyatt, G., Van Zanten, S., Feeny, D. & Patrick, D. (1989) Measuring quality of life in clinical trials: a taxonomy and review. *Canadian Medical Association Journal*, **140**, 1441–8.

Headache Study Group of University of Western Ontario (1986) Predictors of outcome in headache patients presenting to family physicians. *Headache*, **26**, 285–94.

Hope, T., Sprigings, D. & Crisp, R. (1993) 'Not clinically indicated': patients' interests or resource allocation? *British Medical Journal*, **306**, 379–81.

Hunt, S., McEwen, J. & McKenna, S. (1985) Measuring health status: a new tool for clinicians and epidemiologists. *Journal of Royal College of General Practitioners*, **35**, 185–8.

Jenkins, C.D. (1992) Assessment of outcomes of health intervention. *Social Science and Medicine*, **35**, 367–76.

Kahneman, D. & Varey, C. (1991) Notes on the psychology of utility. In: *Interpersonal Comparisons of Well-being* (eds J. Elster & J. Roemer), pp. 127–63. Cambridge University Press, Cambridge.

Kaplan, R. & Anderson, J. (1988) The quality of well-being scale: rationale for a single quality of life index. In: *Quality of Life: Assessment and Application* (eds S. Walker & R. Rosser), pp. 51–77. MTP Press, Leicester.

Kaplan, S., Greenfield, S. & Ware, J. (1989) Impact of the doctor–patient relationship on the outcomes of chronic disease. In: *Communicating with Medical Patients* (eds M. Stewart & D. Roter), pp. 228–45. Sage, London.

Kaplan, R., Anderson, J., Wu, A. *et al.* (1989) The quality of well-being scale: applications in AIDS, cystic fibrosis and arthritis. *Medical Care*, **27**, S27–43.

Kreitler, S., Chaitchnik, S. *et al.* (1993) Life satisfaction and health in cancer patients, orthopedia patients and healthy individuals. *Social Science & Medicine*, **36**, 547–66.

Lefcourt, H. (1981) *Health Locus of Control Scales. Research with the Locus of Control Construct.* Academic Press, New York.

McGee, H., O'Boyle, C., Hickey, A. *et al.* (1991) Assessing the quality of life of the individual: the SEIQoL with a healthy and a gastro-enterology unit population. *Psychological Medicine*, **21**, 749–59.

McGuire, A., Henderson, J. & Mooney, G. (1988) *The Economics of Health Care.* Routledge, London.

Mooney, G. (1992) *Economics, Medicine and Health Care.* Harvester, London.

Najman, J. & Levine, S. (1981) Evaluating the impact of medical care and technologies on the quality of life: a review and critique. *Social Science & Medicine*, **15F**, 107–16.

Newman, S., Fitzpatrick, R., Lamb, R. & Shipley, M. (1989) The origins of depressed mood in rheumatoid arthritis. *Journal of Rheumatology*, **16**, 740–4.

Nord, E. (1991) EuroQol: health related quality of life measurement. Valuations of health states by the general public in Norway. *Health Policy*, **18**, 25–36.

O'Boyle, C., McGee, H., Hickey, A. *et al.* (1992) Individual quality of life in patients undergoing hip replacement. *The Lancet*, **339**, 1088–91.

Orth-Gomer, K. & Uden, A. (1987) The measurement of social support in population surveys. *Social Science & Medicine*, **24**, 83–91.

Pearlman, R. & Uhlmann, R. (1988) Quality of life in chronic diseases: perceptions of elderly patients. *Journal of Gerontology*, **43**, 25–30.

Potts, S. (1992) The QALY and why it should be resisted. In: *Philosophy and Health Care* (eds E. Mathews & M. Menlowe), pp. 44–63. Avebury, Aldershot.

Regan, J., Yarnold, J., Jones, P. & Cooke, N. (1991) Palliation and life quality in lung cancer: how good are clinicians at judging treatment outcome? *British Journal of Cancer*, **64**, 396–400.

Rosser, R. & Kind, P. (1976) A scale of valuations of states of illness: is there a social consensus? *International Journal of Epidemiology*, **7**, 347–58.

Rudick, R., Miller, D., Clough, J. *et al.* (1992) Quality of life in multiple sclerosis: comparison with inflammatory bowel disease and rheumatoid arthritis. *Archives of Neurology*, **49**, 1237–42.

Sackett, D. & Torrance, G. (1978) The utility of different health states as perceived by the general public. *Journal of Chronic Diseases*, **31**, 697–704.

Schag, A., Heinrich, R. & Ganz, P. (1984) Karnofsky performance status revisited: reliability, validity and guidelines. *Journal of Clinical Oncology*, **2**, 187–93.

Schumacher, M. Olschewski, M. & Schulgen, G. (1991) Assessment of quality of life in clinical trials. *Statistics in Medicine*, **10**, 1915–30.

Sensky, T. & Catalan, J. (1992) Asking patients about their treatment. *British Medical Journal*, **305**, 1109–10.

Silberfarb, P., Maurer, H. & Grouthamel, C. (1980) Psychosocial aspects of neoplastic disease I: functional status of breast cancer patients during different treatment regimens. *American Journal Psychology*, **137**, 450–5.

Slevin, M., Plant, H., Lynch, D. *et al.* (1988) Who should measure quality of life, the doctor or the patient? *British Journal of Cancer*, **57**, 109–12.

Smith, A. (1987) Qualms about QALYs. *The Lancet*, **i**, 1134–6.

Spitzer, W., Dobson, A., Hall, J. *et al.* (1981) Measuring the quality of life of cancer patients. *Journal of Chronic Diseases*, **34**, 585–97.

Sprangers, M. & Aaronson, N. (1992) The role of health care providers and significant others in evaluating the quality of life of patients with chronic disease: a review. *Journal of Clinical Epidemiology*, **45**, 743–60.

Stewart, A., Greenfield, S., Hays, R. *et al.* (1989) Functional status and well-being of patients with chronic conditions. *Journal of the American Medical Association*, **262**, 907–13.

Sutherland, H., Lockwood, G. & Boyd, N. (1990) Ratings of the importance of quality of life variables: therapeutic implications for patients with metastatic breast cancer. *Journal of Clinical Epidemiology*, **43**, 661–6.

Teske, K., Daut, R. & Cleeland, C. (1983) Relationships between nurses' observations and patients' self reports of pain. *Pain*, **16**, 289–96.

Uhlmann, R. & Pearlman, R. (1991) Perceived quality of life and preferences for life-sustaining treatment in older adults. *Archives of Internal Medicine*, **151**, 495–7.

Viney, L. & Westbrook, M. (1981) Psychological reactions to chronic illness-related disability as a function of its severity and type. *Journal of Psychosomatic Research*, **25**, 513–23.

Weinberger, M., Hiner, S. & Tierney, W. (1986) Improving functional status in arthritis: the effect of social support. *Social Science and Medicine*, **23**, 899–904.

Wells, K., Stewart, A., Hays, R. *et al.* (1989) The functioning and well-being of depressed patients: results from the medical outcomes study. *Journal of the American Medical Association*, **262**, 914–9.

Williams, A. & Kind, P. (1992) The present state of play about QALYs. In: *Measures of the Quality of Life* (ed. A. Hopkins), pp. 21–39. Royal College of Physicians, London.

Commentary on Chapter 15

Martyn Evans

Fitzpatrick neatly captures a central oddness in the standard utilitarian approach to outcome measures in health care by noticing, first, that (on the best evidence) patients do not agree with the negative valuations placed upon their health states by other people who do not suffer from the illnesses in question; and second, that this seems either not to have occurred to or not to trouble the proponents of that standard outcome measure, the quality adjusted life year (QALY). He concludes that modifications to the QALY's scope could make it sensitive to important dimensions of health care currently (and woefully) ignored in outcome measurement: 'By this means a health care system that is truly patient-centred will emerge'.

Fitzpatrick's key distinction

Fitzpatrick's prescription for developing health care evaluation relies on distinguishing the 'supportive' functions of health care, in effect, those which contribute to the patient's sense of empowerment, assurance and control rather than to survival or to physically symptomatic quality of life. Judging how far this distinction can actually be made and defended will guide us in assessing his prescription.

'Health-related' versus other aspects of quality-of-life

Fitzpatrick takes a somewhat ambivalent view towards a *prior* distinction – that between those components of health care which are 'health-related' and those which by contrast are 'not relevant to health care'. Such a distinction is of course at the mercy of rival definitions of health; the notorious World Health Organization definition would make the distinction empty, hence meaningless. But without such a stultifyingly inclusive notion of health one might still be sceptical as to whether any exclusive subset of contributors to our quality of life can be tied to health. As Fitzpatrick notes, it is not easy to specify health-related quality of life as a 'sub-set of the broader range of personal experience'. On the other hand in arguing *for* the inclusion in health care outcomes, of social as distinct from symptomatological dimensions of patients' quality of life, he seems to promote an emphasis on the former in order to displace the latter. Can we convincingly do this if we cannot clearly distinguish these two dimensions?

'Health status' functions versus 'supportive' functions of health care

Fitzpatrick regards it as obvious that health care is meant to do many other things 'besides improving health status in terms of survival and quality of life', whether or not these other things directly influence health status: 'To regard functions such as reassurance and social support as less relevant to health is arbitrarily to redefine into limbo the activities of most of primary care and much of hospital care'. Putting it thus is, admittedly, somewhat empirical rather than conceptual (and economists warn us against thinking that the purpose or rationale of an institution can be discerned by identifying that institution's typical activities).

Again, Fitzpatrick expends considerable energy on showing how weak is the correlation between physical symptoms and the subjective experience of quality of life construed more broadly; moreover he evidently regards health care's supportive functions as addressing the 'personal satisfactions of [patients'] health care goals'. It is in this light that we want to know why patients value health care's 'supportive' functions. It seems artificial to emphasize such beneficial effects and then to distinguish them as having only functions other than improving health status in the sense defined. It would be better to represent what Fitzpatrick takes to be division of function as instead simply the complexity of both the idea of 'health status' and the project of caring for patients.

Implications of Fitzpatrick's key distinction for outcome measurement

Were we to take the distinction at its face value, and to supplant the emphasis on the mechanical with an emphasis on the 'supportive' as Fitzpatrick recommends, then a revision of our outcome measures would clearly be indicated. None know better than patients how they feel and what is important to them. What kind of revision should this be?

Two broad approaches identified

Fitzpatrick contrasts two kinds of approach to the evaluation of health care. One approach, which he favours, assesses the experiential impact of health care upon the patient, and looks to the patient to define the outcomes to be measured. However he notes that the dominant approach in health economics is quite unlike this; broadly, it regards varying health states as a variety of utilities, whereby the impact of health care is judged in terms of its transferring patients from one quality-adjusted health state to another. The quality of life adjustments, in this tradition, express health states by reference to a narrow, primarily mechanistic set of parameters tied to physical function; such parameters ignore the wider contributors to our quality of life. Worse still they express, not what patients themselves say about what it is *actually* like to be in a certain health state, but what others imagine it *would* be like in the narrow terms described.

A moral or a conceptual case for change?

It might be that the trouble with QALYs is that they simply express the 'wrong' side of Fitzpatrick's key distinction, that is to say the results of the mechanical instead of the 'supportive' functions of health care (and that they do this simply because they ask the wrong people). Here, Fitzpatrick would be making a moral case for changing the ingredients of an essentially unchanged formula. This is confirmed by his concluding conjecture that, with the right amendments to the ingredients, patient-centred care might 'record favourable impacts in utilitarian terms'. He thinks the strongest objection to this is that proponents of QALYs would think it counter-intuitive to trade off life-saving services in favour of more supportive services. This seems to me to deny the first premise of QALYs: namely that sheer survival may on occasion be traded against improved quality of life.

Proponents of QALYs would presumably claim to take our value-preferences as they find them, and simply to maximize whatever these happen to be. Fitzpatrick should, perhaps, have noticed that Williams and Kind's cited objection to a wider scope for QALYs relies on a narrowly and improperly prescriptive notion of suffering. When (he records) they claimed that under such an enlarged view of health care 'People on average will both die sooner and suffer more than they need have done', they forget the tradeability of survival and they define suffering in narrowly physical terms. Fitzpatrick's evidence for a wider conception of suffering amongst patients themselves suggests that what is wrong with QALYs is their conception of quality of life and not simply their too-limited applicability. Hence the real change needed is a conceptual rather than a simply moral one.

Conclusions

Any resource criterion will be used to prioritize patients or patient groups; none can be morally neutral. A patient-centred criterion would have at any rate the moral authority that it approximated what patients themselves distinguished as better and worse effects of health care. Any putative resource criterion has to compete with other candidates. In this sense, patient-centredness is both an embodiment of a certain conception of health, of health states, and of health care, and also a moral claim to be defended on its own terms against other conceptions of good or just health care provision.

Acknowledgement
I am grateful to Dr Tony Hope for suggestions regarding an earlier draft of this commentary.

Index